How to Live with Male & Female Menopause

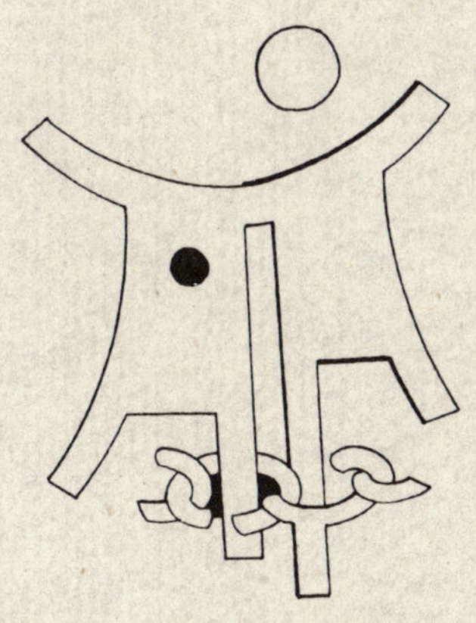

How to Live with Male & Female Menopause

L. C. Gupta M.D. D.Sc (Hon)
Abhishek Gupta M.D., DNB.

Srishti
PUBLISHERS & DISTRIBUTORS

Srishti Publishers & Distributors
64-A, Adhchini
Sri Aurobindo Marg
New Delhi 110 017
srishtipublishers@yahoo.com

First published by Srishti Publishers & Distributors in 2006

ISBN 81-88575-52-6

Typeset in AGaramond 11pt. by Suresh Kumar Sharma at Srishti

Cover design by Sandip Sinha
Email: sundeepsinha@yahoo.co.in

Printed and bound in India

Dedicated to
honourable Mr Suresh Pachauri who
encourages honesty and creativity.

Contents

Section I

FEMALE MENOPAUSE

Preface

Menopause has come to an age. It is now discussed freely by women both at places of work and in many social gatherings. Women are beginning to understand that there is more to the called 'change of life' than simply the cessation of periods. Women wants to know about what happens to their bodies at the time of menopause. They want to know its remedy. They understand that health is more than the absence of disease and are keen to invest time to maintain physical, sexual, emotional and spiritual health.

Estrogen deficiency leads to menopause in females while androgen deficiency leads to new concept of 'male menopause' termed not heard even by many physicians.

Andropause is a term applied to late 50s and beyond where testosterone levels seem to decline causing a variety of symptoms including less of strength, poor sexual functioning, muscle weakness, depressed mood, lower bone destiny and low sex drive. It can be treated up to some extent like its female equivalent with hormone replacement therapy.

Present series of books have been prepared under the aegis of Shakuntala Devi Multi Therapy Health and Research Foundation.

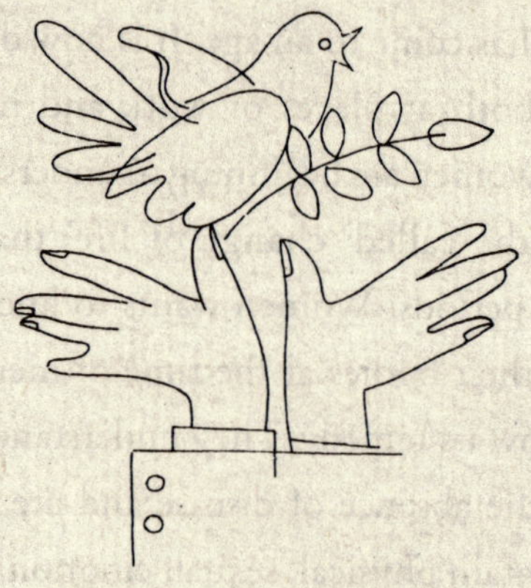

Section I

Female Menopause

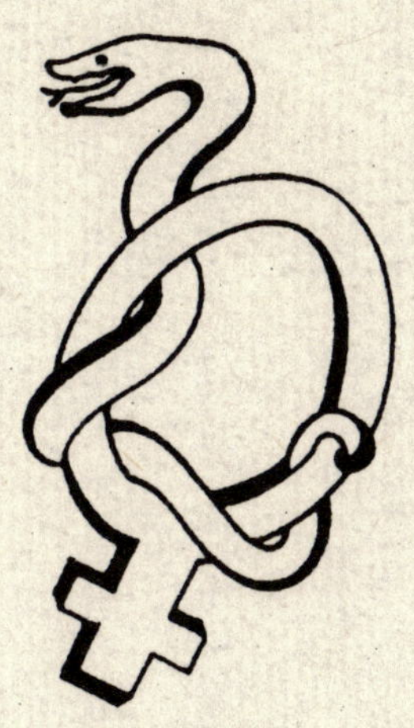

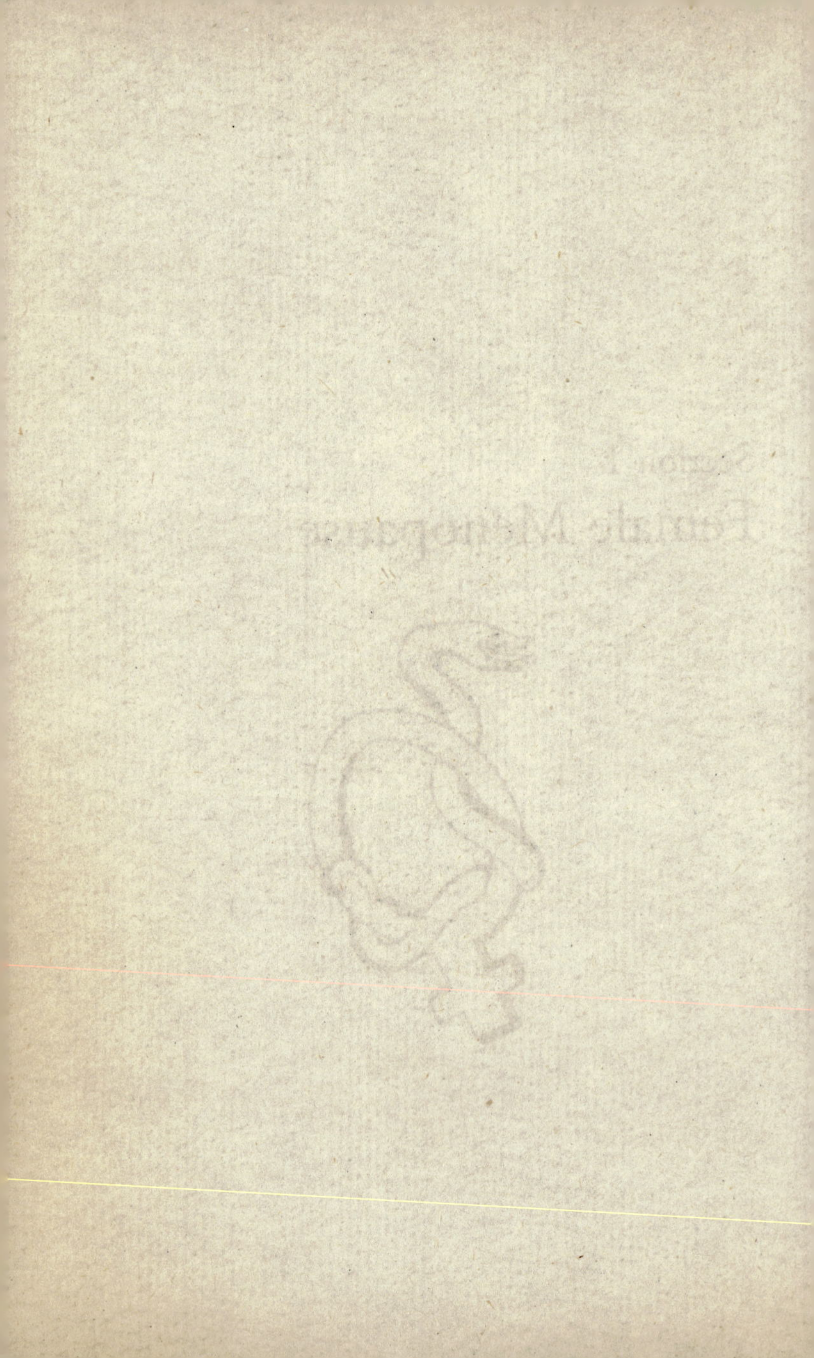

Female Reproductive Organs

Dr. Sujata

Before knowing the menopausal effect on sex behaviour one should know the anatomy and physiology of female sex organs.

What are external genital organs?

The external parts of female genitals visible on the outside of the body and are collectively known as vulva.

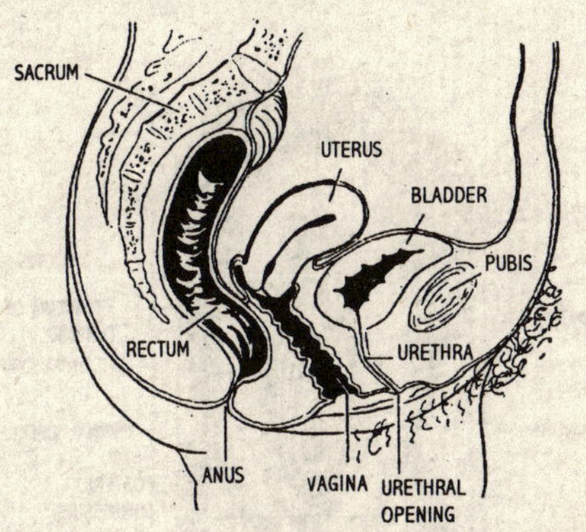

FEMALE REPRODUCTIVE ORGANS

Outer lips are known as labia majora. These are covered by hair. These are formed very irregularly similar to thick, fleshy lips of a tropical flower.

What are inner lips?

It is a set of lips inside. These are thinner, smooth and silky. When sexually aroused these glisten with moisture. These inner lips often curve out and over the outer lips producing a shape like conch shell.

Colour of outer and inner lips includes shades of violet, dusky, crimson, gold and bluish. Outer lips are darker.

What is the role of clitoris?

Most sensitive clitoris lies at the upper end of vagina between the folds of labia. Its glans projects like a pea.

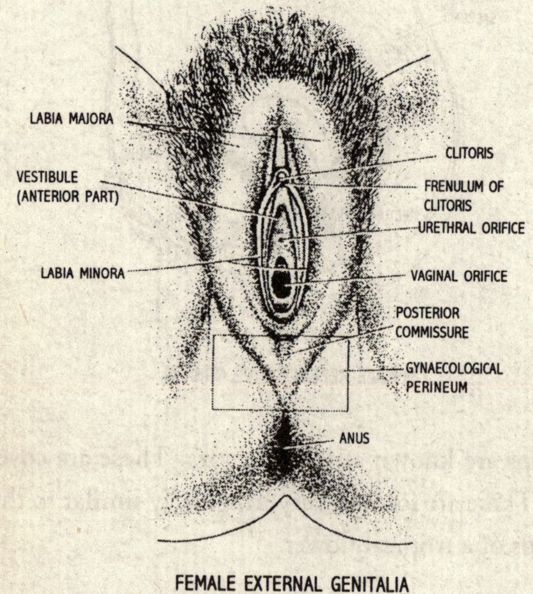

FEMALE EXTERNAL GENITALIA

Many of old men would not have seen this. But if you slip a finger down a little further to the enterance of vagina and press it inward you can feel a root of clitoris. When sexually excited it becomes engorged and thicker.

What is the response of clitoris in the coital act?

During excitement phase both the glans and shaft of the clitoris becomes congested. Glans of clitoris becomes double of its size.

During the plateau phase entire clitoris is retracted under the clitoral hood and disappears from view.

During orgasm the clitoris remains hidden from view. Following an orgasm it quickly re-emerges from its retracted position. When orgasm has not occured the engorgement of the glans and shaft of clitoris may persist for hours and cause discomfort.

What is the role of vagina?

It is a hollow muscular passage. The physiological response of vagina and penis to sexual stimulation are complementary. As penis prepares for penetration the vagina prepares to receives it. Only outer 1/3 of vagina is having nerve endings making it a sensitive part.

During excitement phase there develops 3 specific reactions in vagina –

(i) expansion of inner part.

(ii) lubrication.

(iii) change of colour.

Moistening of vaginal wall is the first sign of sexual response. Lubricatory function is of a clear and slippery vaginal fluid. This fluid is alkaline and tones down the acidity of vagina. On excitement stretched walls of vagina looses some of normal wrinkled appearance. Due to increased blood supply ordinary purple red vaginal walls take on a darker hue.

What happens to the vagina during orgasm?

The area contracts rhythmically at an interval of 0.8 seconds from 6-12 times. After the first 3-6 contractions the movements become weaker and more widely spread. The orgasmic pattern varies from one person to another and in the same person from one orgasm to another.

How breasts respond to sexual act?

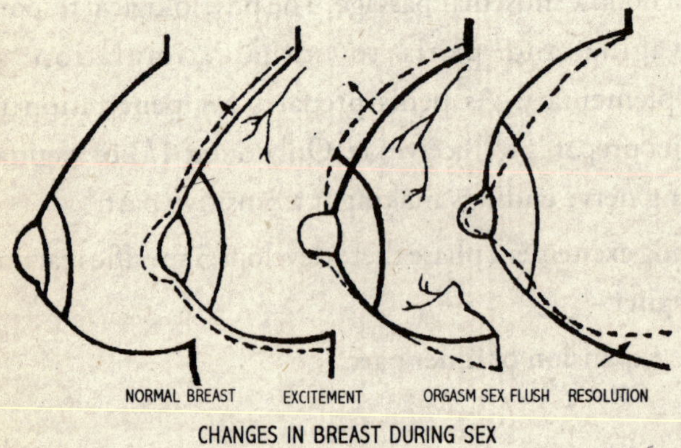

CHANGES IN BREAST DURING SEX

Males also respond to the sexual stimulation. Females do respond better. It happens due to involuntary muscle fibres than vascular congestion. Enlargement of blood vessels is responsible for enlargement of breast as whole including areola.

Changes in the male breasts are inconsistent and restricted to nipple erection. Male nipples are rarely stimulated directly by females.

In the plateau phase the engorgement of areola is more marked. As a result nipples appear smaller. Breasts expand further. During orgasms the breasts show no further changes and after orgasm breasts return to normal size.

What about uterus?

It is shaped like a pear or fig with the stalk tilted down into your vagina. The cramps which are often felt during period are simply tightenings of uterus. During strong orgasm your uterus may also contract. During pregnancy uterus contracts regularly as a kind of rehearsal for birth. Uterus also contracts when breasts are stimulated may even be during breast feeding.

What is the role of ovaries?

Each ovary is about the size and shape of an almond in its shell. If one is not working other takes the work. During the part of reproductive life woman produces a ripe egg, an ovum, every month – usually about two weeks before her next menstrual cycle. During average woman's reproductive life it may occur more than 300 times.

Ovaries manufacture the hormones estrogen and progesterone. Both are steroids.

(i) Estrogen plays a major role in a woman's body in all the physical changes of puberty, menstruation and pregnancy. It is produced every month by ripening egg follicle and levels change at different times in cycle.

(ii) Progesterone is also secreted in a monthly rhythm. It is important in ovulation the rebuilding of the lining of uterus when a period is over and in enriching the wall of uterus to offer nourishment for a fertilized ovum to feed on.

What about the production of estrogen and progesterone?

At the end of menstrual period the estrogen level rises, reaching at peak just before ovulation. Estrogen stimulates the cervix to secrete mucus which is at first thick, sticky and opaque but which gradually changes to become thin, slippery, clear and stretchy like raw white egg. When mucus is like this it allows sperm to swim easily through up into cervix and from there into the uterus and fallopian tube.

After ovulation the level of estrogen drops steeply. Progesterone thickens mucus again to form a plug in the cervix until the next period starts with menstruation.

Primary Amenorrhoea

Dr. Abhitabh

How to define primary amenorrhoea?

Most girls will start menstruating before the age of 15. If menstruation does not start by then, it is known as primary amenorrhoea while secondary sexual characteristics are normal. If there has been no secondary sexual development it is known as delayed puberty.

What is the commonest cause of primary amenorrhoea?

It is most commonly caused by imperforate hymen. The menstrual blood remains in vagina. It causes cylical lower abdominal pain. Rarely there may be horizontal vaginal septum.

There may be family history of delayed menstruation. In such cases norethisterone 5 mg may be given orally for 5 days.

What are the causes of delayed menarche?

Generally girls start their menstruation at the age of 13. Factors which delay a particular level of minimum weight of a teenager, may delay the age of the menarche such as

- Malnutrition.
- Slow growth after birth.
- Premature child.

- Twins.
- Atheletic training.
- Environmental and social factors.

What is secondary amenorrhea?

Secondary amenorrhoea means cessation of established menstruation. In absence of pregnancy if there is no menstruation for 6 months it is known as secondary amenorrhea.

What are the physiological causes of secondary amenorrohea?

Commonest cause of it during reproductive life is pregnancy and lactation. High level of prolactin associated with suckling suppresses ovulation and gives rise to lactation amenorrhea.

Menstrual Cycle

Dr. Sujata

What is menstrual cycle?

In reproductive age group females have menstrual bleeding every month except when she becomes pregnant.

Human beings have monthly cycle while sheep ovulates once a year and rabbit ovulates in response to coitus. Average duration of menstruation cycle is 28 days. Cycle has 3 phases

(i) Follicular phase

(ii) Ovulation

(iii) Post ovulatory or luteal phase.

What is a follicular phase, (days 1-8)?

At the start of the cycle follicular stimulating hormone and luteinizing hormone are relatively high and these stimulate development of 10-20 follicles. Out of which one becomes dominant follicle. Dominant follicle appears during the mid follicular phase. While other follicles undergo atresia.

During and just after the menses estrogen levels are relatively low but they begin to increase as follicular development occurs.

What happens during 9-14 days of follicular stage?

As follicle increases in size it develops a fluid filled central cavity called antrum. It transform a primary follicle into Graffian follicle. There is a increase in production of estrogen and reaches at peak 18 hours prior to ovulation.

What is ovulation, (Day 14)?

It is associated with enlargement of follicle followed by protrusion from the surface of ovarian cortex and then rupture of follicles. Extrusion of oocyte takes place. Certain females can experience a short lived pain in one or both iliac fossa.

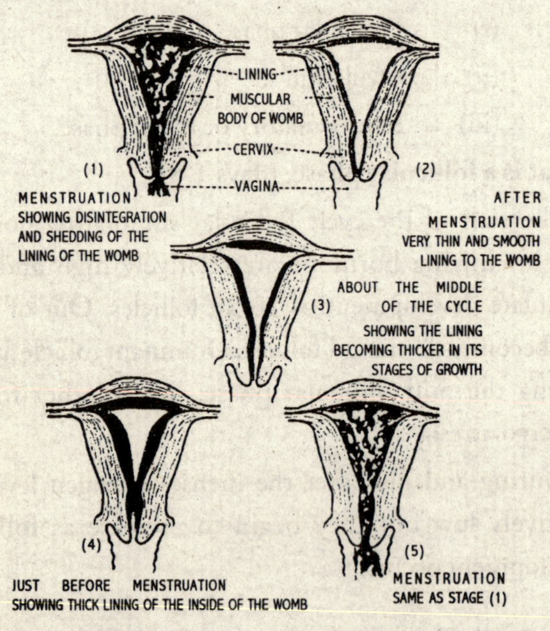

WOMB SHOWING STAGES IN THE MENSTRUATION CYCLE

What happens in luteal phase, 15-28 days?

During this phase granulosa cells undergo luteinizing process and these structures collectively form the corpus luteum. This is the major source of sex steroid hormones, estrogen and projesterone in post ovulatory phase.

If conception and implantation occurs corpus leteum does not regress otherwise it starts regressing on 26-28 days.

What happens in menstrual phase?

Normally luteal phase lasts for 14 days. At the end of it regression of corpus leuteum is associated with a decline

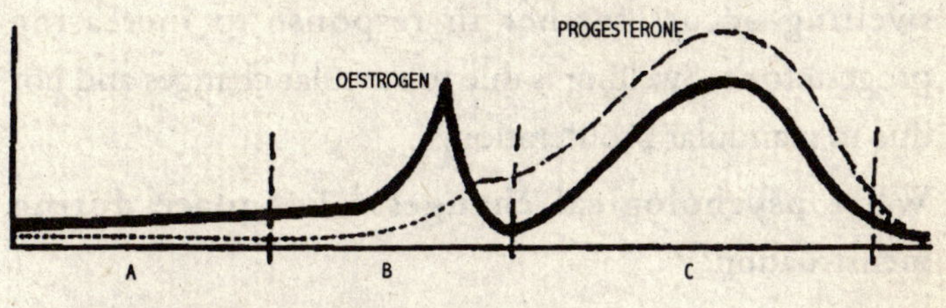

A. MENSTRUAL CYCLE
B. 10 DAYS OF PROLIFERATION PHASE
C. 14 DAYS OF SECRETARY PHASE

HORMONE LEVELS DURING CYCLE

in estrogen and progesterone production. The fall is followed by intense spasmodic contraction giving rise to ischemic necrosis. There will be shedding of superficial layer of endometrium in form of bleeding.

Vasospasm appears to be due to production of prostaglandins. Prostaglandins increase uterine contractions at the time of menstrual flow.

Does body temperature rises during menstrual flow?

A rise in body temperature of about 10^0F occurs following ovulation and is sustained until menstruation starts. It is due to thermogenic effect of progesterone acting on hypothalamic level.

What breast changes takes place during menstruation?

Human breasts are very sensitive to estrogen and progesterone. Breast swelling is the first sign in puberty in response to even small increase in ovarian estrogen. Breast swelling occurs further in response to increasing progesterone. Swelling is due to vascular changes and not due to glandular proliferation.

What psychological changes takes place during menstruation?

There may develop change in mood during menstrual cycle with an increase in emotional lability in the late leuteal phase. These may develop due to falling levels of progesterone.

During menstrual cycle which period is known as 'safe period'?

During safe period if you have unprotected sex chances of pregnancy are rare. It includes four days after menstruation and nine days before menstruation.

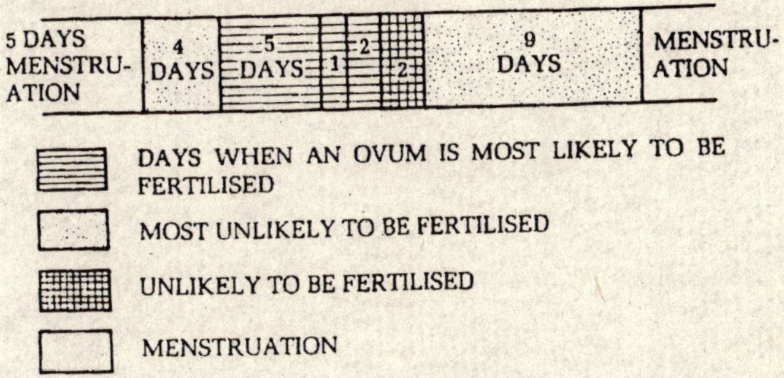

5 DAYS MENSTRU-ATION	4 DAYS	5 DAYS	1	2	2	9 DAYS	MENSTRU-ATION

DAYS WHEN AN OVUM IS MOST LIKELY TO BE FERTILISED

MOST UNLIKELY TO BE FERTILISED

UNLIKELY TO BE FERTILISED

MENSTRUATION

SAFE PERIOD

Premenstrual Syndrome

Dr. Ila Gupta

What is premenstrual syndrome?

It is defined as a regular pattern of symptoms occuring before menstruation with a decreasing of symptoms soon after the bleeding starts. 95% females suffer from mild symptoms.

What are the symptoms of premenstrual syndromes?

A few prominent symptoms include –

- Breast tenderness.
- Headache.
- Oedema.
- Abdominal bloatedness.
- Mood changes.

What is the cause of premenstrual symptoms?

Etiology remains unknown. It may be due to changing patterns of hormones.

What type of pain in breast develops?

Breast pain of PMS is usually cyclical. It is poorly localised and bilateral. Lumpiness is common otherwise non cyclical breast pain is localised and rarely bilateral.

What is the example of a set of diagnostic criteria of PMS?

At least one of the following somatic and affective

symptoms during 5 days before menses in each of three cycles.

Somatic symptoms –

- Breast tenderness.
- Abdominal bloating.
- Headache.
- Swelling.

Affective symptoms –

- Angry outbreaks.
- Depression.
- Irritability.
- Anxiety.
- Confusion.
- Social withdrawl.

Identifiable dysfunction in social or economical performance.

- Discord of relationship confirmed by partner.
- Difficulty in parenting.
- Poor work.
- Increased social isolation.

What are sub groups of PMT?

In 1983 Prof Guy Abraham listed following four sub groups.

(i) PMT – A Characterized by anxiety, irritability and tension.

(ii) PMT – H Weight gain, abdominal bloating.

(iii) PMT – C Increased appetite, fatigue, palpitation and breast pain.

(iv) PMT – D Depressed, withdrawl and suicidal inclination.

How to manage PMS?

It does not require any specific treatment except reassurance. Reducing smoking and drinking may help.

Aerobic exercises leads to increased endorphin levels which improve mood and thus PMS.

How to deal with PMT?

It is associated with high levels of estrogen and low progesterone. Vitamin B_6 in doses of 200-800 mg a day, reduces the estrogen level and increases progesterone and the symptoms. Women should avoid refined sugar and dairy products.

How effect of PMT – H can be reduced?

PMT – H It is characterized by fluid retention. It is associated with high levels of serum testoetone secreted by adrenal glands. Vitamin B_6 in high doses suppresses aldosterone and prevents fluid retention of fluid in tissues. Salt and sugar should be avoided. Spironolactone may also be useful.

How to manage PMT – C ?

It is characterized by food cravings, over eating sweet substances followed by headaches, fatigue and palpitations is associated with increased carbohydrate tolerance and a low level of magnesium. Magnesium improves sugar tolerance and eliminate food cravings.

How to deal PMT – D ?

It is characterized by depression, insomnia and forgetfulness. There may be excessive hair growth. Estrogen supplements help.

What is the relationship between PMT and sex?

Sexual desire dwindles towards the end of menstrual month and is regained once the period commences.

Premature Menopause

Dr. Sekhar Jaiswal

It is natural for menopause to occur naturally after the age of 45 but when it occurs before the age of 40. It is known as premature men.

What are the causes of premature menopause?

Causes include –

(i) Primary ovarian failure – It occurs when woman fails to menstruate at all and medical tests confirm ovarian failure. It is often associated with genetic disorder.

(ii) Secondary ovarian failure – When woman has menstruated normally but subsequently experiences amenorrhoea due to ovarian failure.

What are the feelings of such woman?

Consequences of an early menopause are greater than with a so called normal menopause. Such women deserve more of psychological and emotional support. Lady feels being cheated by nature.

What are the causes of premature menopause?

(i) Surgery – Main cause is removal of ovaries due to any disease. Symptoms may occur within a short space of time if HRT has not started. Such women require long term HRT otherwise heart disease and early osteoporosis may start.

Can hysterectomy bring down an early menopause?

Removal of uterus without ovaries may also bring forward the expected date of menopause. Such women may ignore any symptoms of menopause. Asymptomatic women may not start HRT and suffer.

Can radiotherapy or chemotherapy bring early menopause?

The risk of ovarian failure as a result of radiotherapy depends on age of an individual, dose of radiation and duration of treatment.

Chemotherapeutic agents at the age of around 30 may result in ovarian failure and early menopause.

What are natural or spontaneous cases?

(i) Genetic factor – In Turner's syndrome ovaries develop naturally in utero but accelerates follicular atresia causing ovarian failure.

(ii) Infection like mumps can cause damage to ovaries.

(iii) Addison's disease, diabetes mellitus and hypothyroidism may result in premature ovarian failure.

Do such woman need psychological support?

It can be very traumatic for a woman to know that she has undergone premature menopause when she was eager to have children. She is left unprepared and anxious.

Menopause

Dr. Sujata

What do you understand by menopause?

Term menopause means last menstrual bleed. It is a permanent cessation of menstruation resulting from the loss of ovarian follicular activity.

What is climetric?

It is a period immediately before the menopause. There are endrocrinological changes. There are endrocrinological, biological or clinical features of approaching menopause. This period continues to first few year after the menopause.

How to define post menopause?

This is the area after first year of menopause till one survives.

When to level premature menopause?

Generally menopause starts between the age of 40 to 52 years. But in rare cases some ladies may develop between 30 to 39 years and is known as premature menopause.

On what factors age of menopause depends?

Studies have shown that there is relationship between mother's and daughter's menopausal age. This is sure that age of menopause does not depends on –

- Use of oral contraceptives.
- Number of pregnancies.

- Age of menarche.
- Race.

What are the potential cause of premature menopause?

The cause of premature menopause includes –

- Turner's syndrome.
- Infection with mump's virus.
- Auto immune disease like Addison's disease, diabetes mellitus, and hypothyroidism.

What is surgical menopause?

Removal of uterus and ovaries is the common cause of a premature menopause.

Pathology of Menopause

Dr. Abhishek

What changes takes place in vulva during menopause?

Changes in vulva are related to age and estrogen deficiency. There is decrease in number and coarsening of texture of pubic hair. The labia majora decreases in size. There becomes loss of elasticity. Squamous cell of carcinoma is more common in post menopausal stage. In Paget's disease grossly vulva appears red and valvety with white patches.

What pathological changes in vagina can develop in post menopausal woman?

With estrogen deficiency the vagina shortens with loss of rugal and becomes pale and friable. Bartholin's glands atrophy making vagina dry. Secretion of lubricant fluid is decreased.

How cervix behaves in menopause?

With menopause the cervix decreases in size with decreased stroma and epithelial atrophy and may become flush with vaginal vault. Cervical stenosis may develop and blood with pus collection may take place. There may develop erosion in cervix. There may be loss of superficial epithelial layers or true ulceration with loss of epithelium and formation of granulation tissue.

In the untreated menopausal woman endometrium is often thin and inactive. It is easily inflammed and may lead to bleeding. In case of bleeding all cases should be investigated for cancer.

How myometrium behaves?

The size of uterus decreases with menopause bringing the corpus/cervix ratio from 2:1 to 1:1. Uterine weight decreases in size as low as 30-50 grams while normal weight is 100 gram. Even if uterine fibroids are present, it decreases in size. Uterine vessels often show atherosclerotic changes.

How follopian tubes behaves in menopause?

The fallopian tubes are estrogen target tissues. There is decrease in tubal length and diameter due to atrophy.

What effect is seen on ovaries?

During puberty 300000 egg cells are present in ovary. By 3 years after the menopause, there is visual depletion of germ cells. Menopausal ovary decreases in size. The stroma becomes fibrotic.

What changes are noted in bladder/urethra?

Atrophy of urogenital mucosa is seen in estrogen deficiency. The risk of urinary outflow obstruction increases with age due to narrowing of distal urethra. There may develop urgency, burning, hesitency, frequency and nocturia. Capacity of urinary bladder decreases.

Do bones are also affected in menopause?

Risk of osteoporosis increases owing to a variety of factors at the menopause due to deficiency of estrogen.

What changes takes place in breast at menopause?

There is a decrease in the size of glands and subcutaneous fat of the breast as well as loss of elasticity. The risk of breast cancer develops.

Hot Flushes

Dr. Sekhar Jaiswal

How common are hot flushes during menopause?

Hot flush is conventionally considered the main clinical menifestation of climacteric developing in 75% Indian females, about 40% consult doctors for their agony.

When hot flushes start?

It may start at any age. The onset may be in the perimenopausal phase in a woman who is still menstruating. More often it is first noticed with the onset of menopause. The length of time for which flushes last is also variable. Some may have for a few months while others may continue for years. Some women never flush at all. Flushing can vary in intensity in same woman. Flushes are slight at one year but severe in next year.

Is there any relationship between social status and hot flushes?

There is also great variation with social class and marital status. Lower middle class tend to be less affected. Single woman were reported to suffer more than married women.

What is the mechanism of hot flush?

The process that causes the blood vessels in the surface of skin to dilate is similar to the mechanism that makes us feel hot with embarrassment. But the menopausal hot flush is not the same as blush although both may be precipated or exacerbated by stress.

Does skin temperature rise?

According to J. Jins being yes, but is forgotten that cutaneous temperature reflects the difference between the heat lost to the environment by convection, evaporation, radiation and conduction and that conveyed to the skin by incoming arterial blood. So if rise in skin temperature is to be considered a valid index of rate of flow, the amount of heat lost also become important. Sweating is very common factor raising skin temperature.

Is skin temperature of reliable value?

At high rates of blood flow, skin temperature is thus an insensitive and unreliable indicator of change in local circulation.

Does hot flush is basically a vascular phenomenon.

Yes if we want to know what is happening during the flush it becomes essential to measure, what is happening to blood flow directly. The onset of symptoms of hot flush is associated with an immediate and rapid increase in hand flow which reaches peak in about 3 minutes and remains elevated for 2 minutes. Pulse rate also increases.

Is there any change in blood pressure during hot flush?

No there is no change in blood pressure during period of altered peripheral blood flow and pulse rate. So there is no generalised vasodilator otherwise BP. would have fallen down.

Are hot flush specific to females only?

No, after removal of testis or administration of gonadotropin releasing hormone agonist man may also flush and their symptoms can as severe as in menopausal women. Man will also show a significant rise in both forearm flow and pulse rate.

Are 'flush' and 'blush' the same?

Hot flush is a reflex phenomenon which differs from that observed in response to stress. During hot flush forearm flow rises, a little rise in pulse rate but not associated with rise in BP. In emotional blush blood pressure also rises. Hence flush is therefore not a blush and the flush is not a response to stress.

Are menopausal females more tolerant of heat?

Woman who flush frequently is more intolerant of heat than woman who don't flush. Heat intolerance is present even when they are not flushing.

Are hormones responsible for hot flushes?

Attempts have been made to find out hormonal change in the genesis of flushing. But no one hormone has been found out to be responsible. There are no acute changes in estrogen level before and after flush episode.

Can β-blockers be helpful in menopausal flushing?

No, not at all. It does not reduce the frequency or intensity of hot flushes. Clonidine of α agonist has been used to relieve it.

Breasts in Menopause

Dr. Sujata

What is the anatomy of breast?

Mammary glands lie on both sides on pectoralis muscles. This extends on chest from second rib to 6th rib. Laterally they extend into apical area.

The areolar region contains an elevated nipple through which the primary ducts open. There are 15-20 openings into the nipple. The nipple contains nerves, elastic tissue and muscle which participate in the erectile pattern.

What changes menopause results in breasts?

Estrogen and progesterone secretions and related cellular response decreases slowly from the age of 30 and rapidly after the age of 40.

There develops initial loss of subcutaneous fat and connective tissues followed by degeneration of duct system. Overlying skin becomes thinner, wrinkled and dry. Nipple loses some of the vascularity and becomes light pink instead of red in fair coloured lady.

Firmness of breast is lost.

Are benign breast diseases common after menopause?

After menopause rate of benign tumors of breasts decreases but incidence of malignant tumor increases. One should regularly examine her breasts in bathroom as shown in figure.

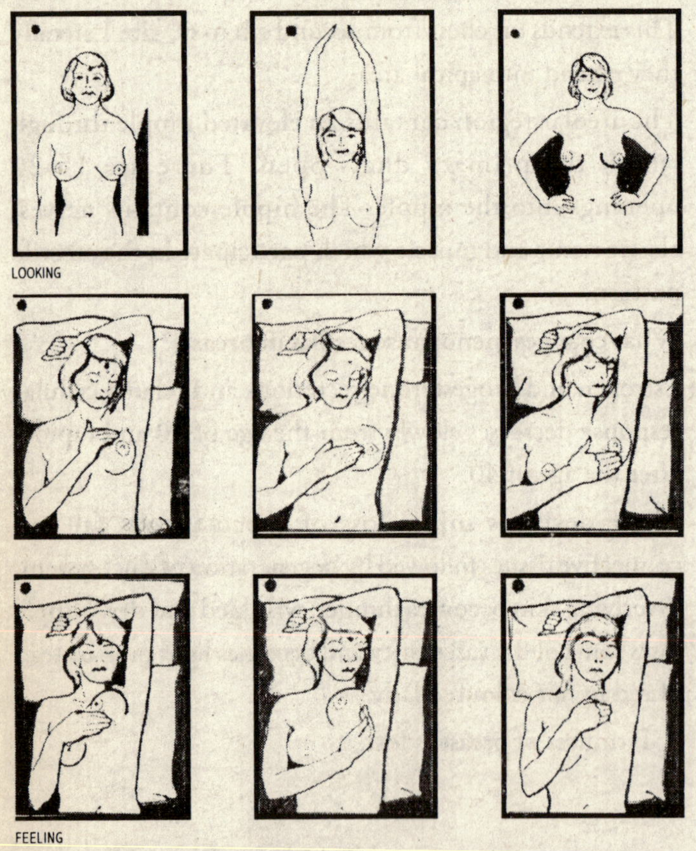

SELF EXAMINATION OF BREASTS TO RULE OUT ANY GROWTH

Nutrition and Menopause

Dr. N. C. Saha

A good healthy diet which is maintained throughout life and especially during menopause will help prevent the occurrence of various diseases.

The concept of healthy diet goes beyond the importance of avoiding an excessive consumption of fats and carbohydrates.

What are the metabolic changes in the post menopausal woman?

The principal cause of death is cardiovascular disease. Hyperlipidémia, hypertension and obesity are the most important factor. To control it weight has to be controlled. The loss of muscular mass and increased redistribution of peripheral fat in women have the immediate consequence of drop in estrogen production. The problem lies in imbalance between energy ingested and that consumed in metabolic process. The basal energetic requirements diminish by 2% per decade during adult life. If this is not compensated this drop could lead to an increase of 1-1.5 kg in weight per year i.e. 10-15 kg in every decade.

What about the metabolism of calcium?

Plasma calcium level depends on balance between calcium ingested and bone resorption, intestinal absorption and renal tubular resorption on one hand and calcium loss in bone formation on another. During menopause there is a greater deterioration of such balance due to –

- deminished intestinal calcium absorption.
- decrease in 1, 25 dihydroxy-vitamin D.
- diminished ingestion of calcium.
- hypercalciuria.

So, how to overcome this problem?

Alteration in metabolism is perhaps the main risk factor which is to be corrected to prevent osteoporosis in menopause. Foods rich in calcium are the best source of intake.

What are the rich calcium source foods?

Rich sources of calcium gm/100 gram

Food	gm/100 gm	Food	gm/100 gm
Milk cow	0.12	Carrot	0.34
Milk buffalo	0.21	Fish dried	1.8
Cheese	0.79	Sitaphal	0.8
Black gram	0.20	Mint	0.20

daily requirement of calcium is 0.5 gram/day.

How to prevent cardiovascular disease?

Apart from diet, both physical exercise and healthy life style are the axis upon which prevention of cardiovascular disease should turn. Three basic measures include –

- Reduce daily intake of saturated fats less than 7% of total calories and cholesterol less than 200 mg per day.
- Reduce weight.
- Increased physical activity.

What is P/S ratio?

The relationship between polyunsaturated fatty acids and saturated fats can be expressed as P/S index. of the hyperlipidemic capacity of fats. It means that those fats with a P/S index higher or equal to 0.5 are hypercholesterolemic. It confirms that 1 gm. of saturated fat has a double hyperlipidemic power than that of 1 gm. of polyunsaturated fat.

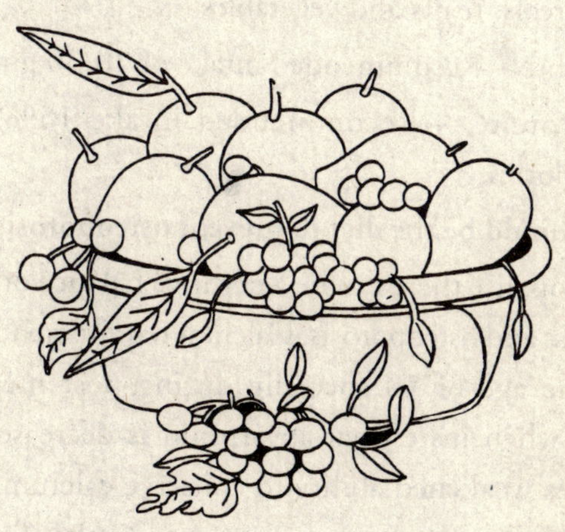

What type of diet should be consumed by menopausal female?

Due to metabolic changes that occur with hypoestrogenism and determine a risk in terms of altered levels of lipoproteins in menopause. Diet should be –

- Polyunsaturated fats – Recommended intake up to 10% of total calories.
- Saturated fats – Recommended intake upto 7% of total calories only.
- Monounsaturated fats – Recommended intake upto 20% of total calories.
- Total fats – Recommended between 25 and 30% of calories.
- Carbohydrate – Total intake 50-60% derived from cereals, fruits and vegetables.
- Fibre – Recommended intake of 20-30 gm/day.
- Proteins – Recommended intake 15% of total calories.

What should be the diet to prevent osteoporosis?

In menopause there can be a negative balance of calcium, bone loss and osteoporosis. Calcium requirement increases after the age of 50 specially during post menopausal period when instestinal absorption is decreased. There becomes weakened ability to conserve calcium. Both of these effects are due to decreased levels of estrogen.

Minimum dietary requirement of this mineral is 1200 mg daily.

Vitamin D (calciferol) is a fat soluble vitamin and fundamental role is to assure the plasmic levels of calcium and phosphates needed for mineralization of bones.

The principal source of vitamin D is ultraviolet rays from sun light. So adequate exposure to sun is needed. This vitamin is also available in fish liver oil, animal fats, egg yolk or supplementary fortified food products. Recommended daily intake of this vitamin is 400 i.u./ day.

It is clear that calcium can reduce bone mineral loss, specially during first five years after menopause and it reduces the incidence of fractures.

What about the nutrition in case of cancer breast?

Countries where soyabean and its bye products are used in plenty, rate of cancer breast is very low during and post menopasual group.

Similary if your fiber consumption is 11.1 gm/day derived from vegetables, fruits cereals and legumes, rate of cancer colon will come down soon.

What is the role of isoflavones?

Some isoflavone supplements have been shown to be effective by improving levels of high density lipoprotein (HDL). Daily intake of 25 gram of soya protein is a dietary complement in low saturated fat and low cholesterol diets reducing the risk of coronary disease.

In what doses isoflavones will be useful?

- The maximum reduction of cholesterol requires about 50 mg daily of isoflavones. FDA has recommended 40-80 mg of isoflavones to obtain arterial compliance. To have effect as antioxident 10 mg daily is needed.
- 50 mg is needed to obtain benefit for bone mass.
- 40-80 mg daily is needed for benefit of vasomotor symptoms.

What is the role of n-3 fatty acids?

Fish contains n-3 fatty acids. Effects of n-3 fatty acids in post menopausal women have been studied with and without hormone replacement therapy, where their actions have proved infuence on cardiovascular factors. It reduces triglycerides and increases HDL.

What about alcohol consumption?

Women are more susceptible to toxic effect of alcohol. In no case they should consume more than 40 gram of ethanol. On the other hand it has been proved that 20 gram of ethanol improves response to insulin by 7% and reduce triglycerides by 10%.

Can certain foods be helpful to relieve hot flushes?

Some ladies get relieved by eliminating caffeine, sugar and alcohol. Vitamin E and B6 also appear in the folklore concerning menopausal symptoms. Evidence is mostly ancedotal.

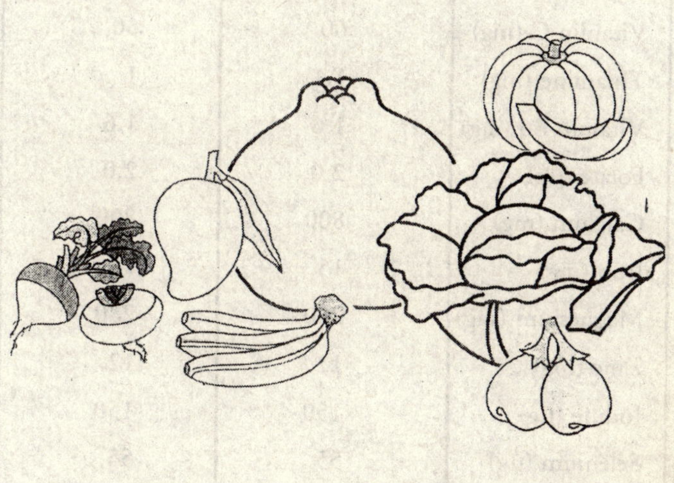

What is a recommended dietary allowance for adult women.

Nutrient	25-50 years	Above 50 years
Vitamin A (μg)	800	800
Vitamin D (μg)	5	5
Vitmin E (mg)	8	8
Vitamin C (mg)	60	60
Thiamine (mg)	1.1	1
Vitamin B6 (mg)	1.6	1.6
Folate (μg)	2.0	2.0
Calcium (mg)	800	800
Iron (mg)	15	10
Magnesium (mg)	280	280
Zinc (mg)	12	12
Iodine (μg)	150	150
Selenium (μg)	55	55

Osteoporosis and Menopause

Dr. Raju Vaishya

Osteoporosis is a major disabling factor at menopause. Osteoporosis is due to an uncoupling of bone formation and resorption. It is a skeletal disorder where bone strength is compromised due to loss of bone density.

How to classify osteoporosis?

(i) Type I primary osteoporosis – It is due to increased osteoclast activity. It is known as post menopausal osteoporosis.

(ii) Type II primary osteoporosis – It is known as osteoporosis due to ageing. Here bone formation lags behind than bone resorption.

(iii) Secondary osteoporosis – Osteoporosis neither menopause nor due to ageing but due to diseases such as Cushing's syndrome or steroids.

What is the pathology of osteopcrosis?

Osteoporosis is characterized by decreased bone formation resulting in increase in resorption and bone loss. Trabecular bone is more affected than cortical bone. Decreased bone formation results from reduced osteoblasts. There is negative calcium balance due to intestinal absorption and increased calcium loss.

Postmenopausal women with significant hyperthyroidism are at greater risk of fracture.

What are the causes of secondary osteoporosis?

Common causes are –

(i) Endocrine –

Hypogonadism.

Cushing's syndrome.

Hyperthyroidism.

Type I diabetes.

(ii) Malignancy –

Multiple myeloma.

Lymphoma.

Leukemia.

(iii) Drugs –

Heparin.

Anticonvulsants.

Vitamin A excess.

Alcohol.

Corticosteroid.

(iv) Immobilization –

Paralysis.

Hip/lumbar fracture

(v) Genetic/others

Rheumatoid arthritis.

Osteogenesis imperfecta.

(vi) Renal –

Renal failure.

Idiopathic Hypercalciurea.

(vii) Gastrointestinal –

Alcohol.

Malabsorption.

Low vitamin D intake.

Loss of appetite.

What are the risk factors of osteoporosis?

Risk factors for osteoporosis are –

- Family history.
- Personal history of non traumatic fracture.
- Late puberty and early menopause.
- Removal of ovaries before the age of 45.
- Sedentary life style.
- No children.
- Excessive alcohol consumption.
- Steroids, thyroid hormone.
- Excessive sweating.

How to classify types of osteoporosis?

Classification of osteoporotic type

Factor	Post meno pausal	Senile	Secondary
Age	50-70	71-85	Any age
Sex ratio	20:1	2:1	1:1
Fracture site	Spine	Hip, pelvis numerus	Hip, spine peripheral
Trabecular	+++	++	+++
Cortical	+	++	+++
Menopause	+++	++	++
Para thyroid hormone	↓	↑	↓↑
Calcium absorption	↓	↓	↓

What is senile osteoporosis?

It occurs in both male and female. Patients present with fractures of hip, pelvis, humerus and vertebra. Malabsorption of calcium is most common. Vitamin D deficiency due to inadequate exposure to sunlight or to low intake of vitamin D and calcium is also common in elderly people who are housebound. This can lead to malabsorption of calcium, secondaryhyperparathyroidism and ostemomalacia. Decreased ability of aging kidney to produce 125 $(OH)_2$ D_3 is another factor responsible for decreased calcium to negative calcium balance, which stimulates parathyroid function which in turn promotes further bone loss.

Low circulating levels of estrogens are also important in developing pathogenesis of type II osteoporosis.

What is the pathophysiology of osteoporosis?

It is mainly associated with spine and colles fracture. It is associated with trabecular bone loss than cortical bone. The mineral density of spine bone in these patients is more than 2 standard deviation low for mean age. Iliac crest bone biopsies show a reduced bone volume and 25% of

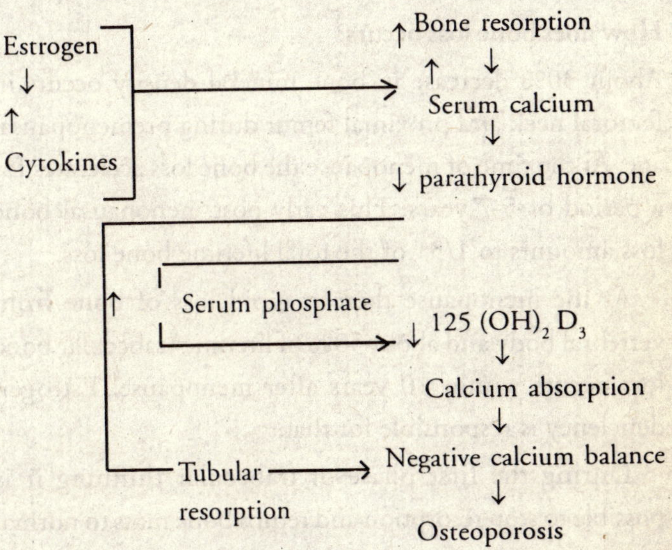

patient shows high bone resorption rate. Bone loss can be 1 to 10% every year for first few years of menopause.

Estrogen deficiency is thought to be the primary cause of menopausal osteoporosis.

What is modelling and remodelling of bone?

Adult skeleton remodels throughout life. It is composed of 60% cortical bone and 20% cacellous i.e. trabecular bone. Process of bone modelling involves both bone formation and resorption, the former exceeding the later. Once initial modelling is complete, bone is then renewed throughout life known as remodelling. During remodelling older bone is replaced and renewed with new bone.

How does bone loss occurs?

About 30% decrease in bone mineral density occurs in femoral neck and proximal femur during premenopausal age. At the time of menopause the bone loss acclerates for a period of 5-7 years. This early post-menopausal bone loss amounts to 1/3rd of the total lifetime bone loss.

At the menopause there is rapid loss of bone from vertebral body and about 50% of litetime trabecular bone loss occurs within 10 years after menopause. Estrogen deficiency is responsible for that.

During the first phase of trabecular thinning it is possible to stop resorption and return bone mass to normal

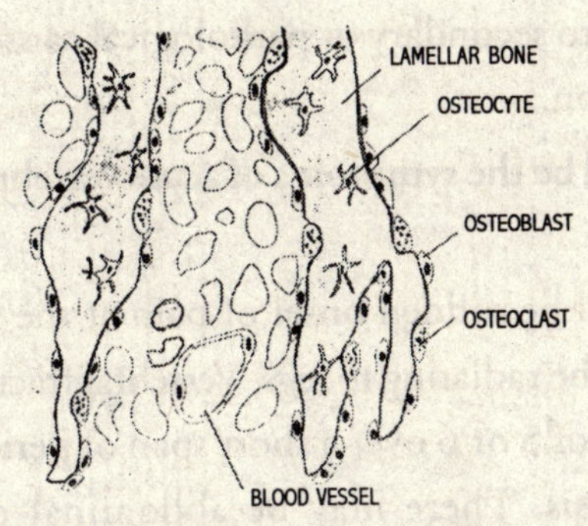

NORMAL BONE

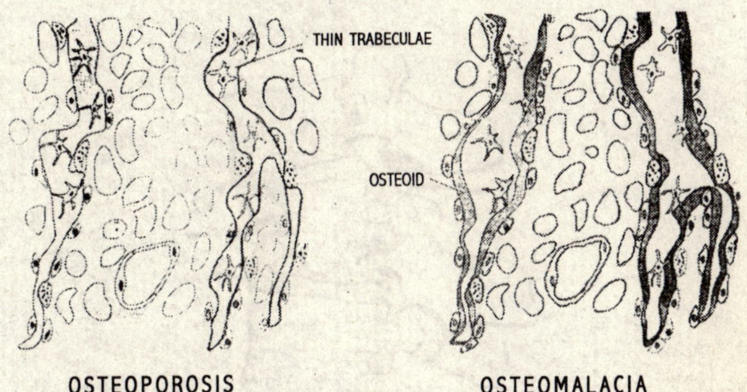

OSTEOPOROSIS OSTEOMALACIA

but in second phase resorptive agents can only prevent further bone loss.

What are the clinical features of osteoporosis?

Vertebral fractures are the commonest type of osteoporotic fracture. These are generally asymptomatic and are diagnosed on routine X-Rays.

Fracture occuring in the cervical or upper thoracic above

T_6 is due to secondary or pathological cause such as tumor or infection.

What will be the symptoms of acute vertebral compression fracture?

There will be sudden onset of pain at the site of fracture. Pain may be radiating to legs. Vertebral fractures may occur in cluster of 5 or 6 over a short span of period. It may lead to kyphosis. There may be abdominal distension and discomfort.

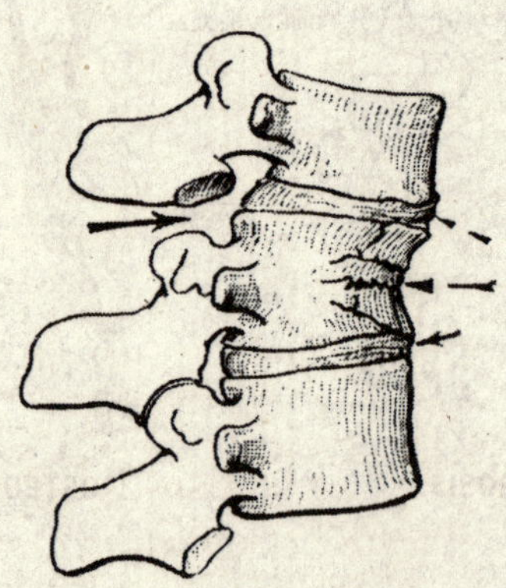

FRACTURE VERTEBRA DUE TO OSTEOPOROSIS

What happens in hip fractures?

Hip fractures are second in frequency. These are always associated with fall, but whether the fracture precedes or follows the fall is not clear. Patient of impacted hip fracture retains the ability to walk but cannot remain stand.

How WHO has defined osteoporosis?

WHO has defined osteoporosis in terms of bone mineral density in post menopausal lady.

Diagnosis	Bone mineral density
Normal	T score ≤ – 1
Osteopenia	T score between – 1 and 2.5
Osteoporosis	T score ≥ 2.5 without fracture
Severe Osteoporosis	T score ≥ 2.5 with a history of fragility fracture.

T score, the number of standard deviations above or below the average bone mineral density value for young healthy woman.

How calcium supplementation helps?

Calcium supplementation alone is not sufficient to prevent either menopausal or age related loss. Toxicity of calcium is kidney-stone formation. Calcium citrate or calcium gluconate are better tolerated. 24 hour urinary calcium should remain within 150-250 mg. Calcium citrate should be avoided because it enhances aluminum absorption and can worsen the bone disease.

Are estrogens helpful in osteoporosis?

Estrogen treatment begun within 5 years of menopause and continued for 10 years reduces hip fractures by 50% and significantly reduces radial and vertebral fractures.

How calcitonin helps?

It is useful in trabecular bone. It prevents hip fractures, utilising calcitonin proves preventive treatment for menopausal trabeculation bone loss. 200 i.u. salmon calcitonin nasal spray reduced the risk of vertebral fracture by 36%.

Draw back of calcitonin therapy is its high cost and need for parentral, nasal or rectal administration. It may develop nausea and vomiting.

Are biophosphates useful?

Biophosphates are used for the prevention and treatment of post menopausal osteoporosis. Recommended dose is 10 mg of alendronate. For prevention 5 mg is sufficient. It is to be taken daily in morning with 225 ml of water. Patient should remain upright and empty stomach for 30 minutes. Calcium supplement 1500 mg/daily will help.

How raloxifene is useful?

Raloxifene has a better favourable therapeutic profile than estrogen. It is an agonist for bone but unlike estrogen is an antagonist for breast and uterine tissue. It is therefore safer than estrogen. It modestly reduces bone turnover and increases BMD and if given 30 mg/day decreases the fracture of spine by 30%.

Can parathyroid hormone be helpful?

Parathyroid hormone given by daily injection is anabolic for skeleton and does not cause bone resorption. It increases BMD by inhibiting bone resorption. It decreases 60% vertebral fractures.

What is the role of vitamin K to reduce the risk of osteoporosis?

Recently it has become evident that vitamin K has a significant role to play in bone health. Greatest source of it is bacteria inhabitating the large bowel. Spinach contains small amount of this vitamin. High dose of vitamin K prevents bone loss, increases bone mass and reduces fracture risk in osteoporotic patients. Vitamin K and vitamin D works together. Vitamin K positively affects calcium balance.

Is prosphorus needed for bone health?

Phosphorus is the second most abundant mineral in bone. Meat, poultry, fish, eggs, legumes and cereals contain phosphorus.

What is the role of sodium in maintaining health of bone?

High sodium diet causes increased urinary calcium losses, as the excretion of sodium is tied to calcium in proximal tubule of kidney. It is estimated that excretion of 1 gm of sodium is associated with loss of about 15 mg of calcium in urine. While we cannot increase sodium consumption due to probable problem of blood pressure we should increase the consumption of calcium.

Mood and Menopause

Dr. Dhananjay Gupta

Relationship of mood changes and menopause continue to be a controversial topic. This period is a period of increased susceptibility of depression and other affective disorder. Psychological changes such as departure of children from home, illness and death of parents, separation or divorces makes this period more confusing.

What is the relationship between gonadal hormones and brain?

Estrogen, progesterone and androgens all have neuroactive and psychoactive properties. Behaviorally estrogen have arousing and antidepressant effect to animal models of depression.

Do beautiful women undergo more of depression during menopause?

It is not being beautiful, but once woman is recognised as beautiful her romance with the self, fame and success starts. She becomes a narcissist who loves only herself and is not capable of loving anyone. She gets a lot of attention and is in a position to pick and choose. Beautiful and successful woman is always on a pedestal and cannot differentiate between fantasy and beautiful. At menopause due to lack of estrogen her face continue to change in manliness. She develops fear of being left by husband. And her mind does not settle for anything that's second best and she starts undergoing depression.

Why breaks up in relationship are more during menopause?

Beauty gives the man an initial high when he is still in process of falling in lust but soon the same beauty start giving convulsions to his ego. It leads to major threats in securities and fear of loosing his woman to a more successful man who is more attractive too. She feels she is above everyone and cannot survive any relationship. During menopause irritation, frustration and hot flushes adds fuel to fire and breaking up starts.

Is infidelity more common in old age and how partner should behave?

All men desire to sleep with other women during their permanent relationship. Whether they act on it or not depends on opportunity, courage and intensity of desire. Very often it is infidelity which breaks us. Because pillar of our relationship was on the sole pillar of fiedelity. But if there are larger, deeper bonds binding couple then despite this crippling blow the relationship will stand not as a symbol of compromise but as an acknowledgement of human fratalities and the strength of love.

Thyroid and Menopause

Dr. Abhishek Gupta

What are the anatomical features of thyroid?

The thyroid gland lies in the anterior portion of trachea. In adult woman it weighs about 12-20 gram and is responsible for extraordinary metabolic activity. During menopause thyroid gland ages.

It consists of two lobes with a thin isthmus in between. Isthmus lies just below the cricothyroid cartilage. Right lobe is generally larger and more vascular. Thyroid is extremely vascular. It is larger in man than in woman.

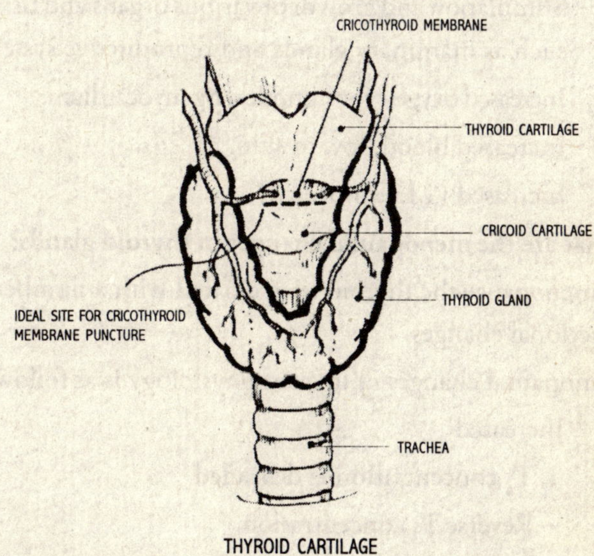

THYROID CARTILAGE

What is the physiology of thyroid hormones?

Thyroid gland secretes thyroxine (T_4) and tri idothyroxine (T_3) All this exist in plasma. T_4 is highest in concentration and arises solely from thyroid gland. T_3 is secreted to a slight extent from thyroid, but most T_3 is obtained from peripheral metabolism by the removal of a single iodine atom from T_4.

What are the functions of thyroid hormones?

- An increase in oxygen consumption.
- An increase in carbohydrate absorption.
- An increase in excretion of cholesterol into biliary tract.
- An increase in lipolysis.
- An increase in basal metobolism.
- Stimulation and growth of various organs and tissues such as mammary glands and reproductive system.
- Increased oxygen consumption by myocardium.
- Increased blood flow to skin.
- Increased G.I.T. motility.

What are the menopausal changes in thyroid glands?

In menopause the thyroid is associated with a number of functional changes.

Menopausal changes in thyroid physiology is as follows –

- Increased

  T_4 concentration is degraded.

  Reverse T_3 concentration.

- Decreased

  Renal iodide clearance.

  T_3 concentration.

  Thyroid iodide clearance.

  Total T_4 production.

What is hypothyroidism?

Hypothyroidism is a condition caused by thyroid failure where there is deficient supply of thyroid hormone available to peripheral tissue.

Prominent clinical features include puffy, face, non pitting oedema.

What are the clinical features of hypothyroidism in menopausal woman?

Symptoms include

- Dry skin.

  Hair loss.

  Cold intolerance.

  Edema of face and eyelids.

- Neurological

  Ataxia.

  Dementia.

- Psychiatric.

  Depression

  Apathy.

Psychosis.

Cognitive dysfunction.

- Musculo skeletal.

  Arthritis.

  Myopathy.

- Metabolic.

  Weight gain.

  Hypercholoesterolemia.

  Peripheral oedema.

- Cardiovascular.

  Pericardial effusion.

  Slow heart.

  Congestive heart failure.

What is thyroidism?

Thyroiditis is much less common in menopausal than in premenopausal women. Thyrotoxicosis may also be produced by toxic multinodular goiter, toxic adenomas and excessive hormone ingestion.

What are the clinical features of hyperthyroidism?

- Cardiovascular symptoms.

  Palpitation.

  Congestive heart failure.

- Psychiatric.
  - Depression.
  - Apathy.
  - Lethargy.
  - Irritability.
- Gastrointestinal.
  - Decreased appetite.
  - Weight loss.
  - Nausea.
  - Constipation.
- Musculoskeletal.
  - Muscle atrophy.
  - Proximal muscle weakness.

What is the line of treatment?

Woman in menopause often do very well with antithyroid medication for 6 months to a year.

Radioactive ablation which is commonly used in menopausal woman may cause some damage to peripheral tissues.

Dyspareunia During Perimenopause

Dr. L. C. Gupta

How to classify sexual pain disorder?

- Dyspareunia – It is a recurrent or persistent pain during sexual intercourse.
- Vaginismus – It is a recurrent or persistent spasm of musculature of outer 1/3 of vagina which interferes with vaginal penetration.
- Non coital sexual pain – Recurrent or persistent genital pain due to non coital sexual stimulation.

What is the frequency of dyspareunia?

Five to ten per cent of fertile and about 40% postmenopausal women complain of various degrees of dyspareunia.

What is the cause of dyspaneunia in perimenopause?

Sexual pain may be felt in introital area or at mid vagina or deep in pelvis.

- Superficial dyspareunia – pain felt superficially.
- Mid vaginal dyspareunia – pain felt at mid vagina.
- Deep dyspareunia – pain felt in deep pelvis.

There may be multiple causes, biological and psychosexual or endocrine.

What are the biological causes of introital and mid vaginal dyspareunia?

Vaginal estrogen concentration may be insufficient for sufficient genital arousal and lubrication. If serum estradiol levels were below 50 µg/ml. there was more dryness, dyspareunia and pain.

What are the leading biological causes of dyspareunia in perimenopause?

Causes include –

- Dyspareunia.
  Lack of sexual hormone.
  Vulvar dystrophy.
  Vulvovaginitis.
- Deep dyspareunia.
  Endometriosis.
  Pelvic inflammatory disease.
  Pelvic variococele.

What is the relationship between vaginitis, vulvitis and dyspareunia?

Vaginitis and vulvitis may be the frequent cofactors of acquired dyspareunia in the perimenopausal years. Normal pH of vagina remains below 4.5. Certain infections are common at higher pH above 5. Loss of estrogen and high pH results in dyspareunia.

How vulvar dystrophy affects?

It is a full thickness disorder. It is not limited to mucocutaneous area. It is probably genetic accelerating hormone receptor loss. It results in difficulty in getting genitally aroused.

What are vascular and metabolic factors?

Smoking, atherosclerosis hypertension and diabetes may all contribute to general arousal disorder resulting in dyspareunia.

Can emotional disharmony may result in dyspareunia?

If there is lack of emotional intimacy, relationship is abusive resulting in dryness of vagina leading to dyspareunia.

How pelvic inflammatory disease leads to dyspareunia?

It may lead to deep pelvic pain. When old females have unprotected sex with new partners may lead such infection.

Can dyspareunia be of life long duration?

If pain prevents penetration there is a possibility of vaginismus. Low libido also may result it.

What is situational dyspareunia?

It may develop due to frustrated intimacy and love needs. There develops loss of libido and arousal disorder.

When pain develops?

Pain before intercourse suggests a phobic attitude towards penetration. Pain during intercourse is frequently reported.

It is mostly due to organic disease. Pain after intercourse suggests vestibulitis.

How to manage dyspareunia?

Testosterone propionate powder 2% in jelly is applied to the external genitalia daily in very small quantity. This increases clitoral arousal, sensitivity and responsiveness. Some therapy to vulva will relieve entetry dyspareunia due to vulvar dystrophy.

Vaginal estrogen offers rapid relief when dyspareunia is more dependent on vaginal dystrophy. Tropical estrogen may be the first line of treatment.

Systemic HRT is indicated in loss of libido and poor central arousal.

Emotional Response to Menopause

Dr. A. K. Saxena

Menopause brings physical and psychological change. Anxiety, misery and minor depression occur at this time.

What social changes takes place during menopause?

At menopause many changes occurs, parents may die, children leave home to other city either for studies or job. The more mature she is more she will be able to adjust to loss and change.

Who is a mature lady?

Mature lady is one who is not much dependent on others and is flexible enough to change aims and goals as per need. This may depend on degree of satisfaction.

What are the other causes of dissatisfaction?

If lady was educated and could not do job being busy in reproduction and looking after the child she feels again the loss of self esteem and great sense of regret over lost career opportunities. She often blames children and husband and may continue to achieve through her children putting extra pressure on them for success. But marriage of male child around this time takes the son away and does not remain under her control. This change may set in depression.

What about females who never became mother.

Just after marriage they never wanted to become pregnant and remained busy in career. And they undergo panic after 40 when they have not had a child. They could not take up the opportunity when it was there.

How the loss of parents affects at menopause?

In more inmature woman loss of parents is experienced more than just sadness. The loss may produce a feeling of panic and a fear of inability to cope. She may express in form of loss of loss of libido and symptoms of anxiety.

How a menopausal woman reacts to arrival of her daughter-in-law?

When marriage is not very successful in terms of happiness woman uses children as an emotional replacement of husband and invest all her good loving feelings in child. The loss of child by his marriage may develop intense feelings of loss and envy towards new comer daughter-in-law, who she is otherwise expected to love.

How a 'single woman' reacts to her menopause?

Such women suffer a least. The reasons may be multifactorial because such women have come to terms gradually over a number of years with non fulfillment of a role female.

Pregnancy in Perimenopausal Women

Dr. Ila Gupta

Now a days pregnancies during perimenopausal are not very common as used to be in past before the invent of condom and employment opportunities for women. On the side by side first pregnancy after the age of 32 is increasing partly because of voluntary delays in conception.

What about fertility in old age?

One should remember that there is an age related decline in the ability to conceive. Male also develops sub fertility. Decreased coital frequency also contribute to the longer intervals between pregnancies.

Studies suggest a 20-30% decline in ability to conceive after the age of 35.

What about spontaneous abortion during perimenopause period?

It is well known that rate of spontaneous abortion increases progressively as maternal age rises. If an old lady becomes pregnant with donated young ova she can continue and deliver pregnancies successfully. It means aging of oocyte plays a great role in continuing of pregnancy.

Are there more fetal defects if perimenopause lady conceives?

The most common trisomes observed in live born children

include down syndrome, trisomy 18 and trisomy 47. 20 years old woman has a risk of 1:2000 of delivering a down syndrome baby, while a 35 year old woman has a risk of 1 in 350.

What are the two common medical complications of pregnancy in old age?

There are two common medical problems noted in old age diabetes and hypertension. 8 to 10% females develop pre eclampsia.

What type of obstetric complications you get in old age?

Malpresentations are very high even 11% in women aged 40. Contributory factors are high parity, prematurity, placental dysfunction and growth restrictions.

Menopause and Female Sexuality

Kusum Gupta

Immediately before and following the menopause, majority of women experience changes in sexual function.

What type of sexual changes takes place in menopause?

It may include decrease in sexual activity, decreased sexual responsiveness and decline in sexual interest.

Why these changes takes place?

Decreased estrogen production appears to be the most significant hormonal change with regard to sexual function along with some ovarian hormones.

What can be the non hormonal factors?

Non hormonal functions include psychological reactions to being menopausal sexual changes in male partner, interpersonal conflicts and social attitude towards sex.

Are there authentic studies about this fact?

Kinsey etal (1953) studied female sexual behaviour throughout life. Forty eight per cent of women reported decrease in coital frequency and coitus leading to orgasm. Pleiffer etal (1972) found that 31% by the age of 56-60 were having 'no intercourse' Hallstrom (1973) also found decline in capacity for orgasm, an increase in dyspareunia and reduced coital activity. Van keep etal (1974) found decrease in sexual activity and decrease in quality of sexual experience.

What about sensation of 'touch' during menopause?

Sexual function is affected by sexual touch perception. Touch avoidance was reported by 11% premenopausal women and 46% in 1-3 year post menopausal group.

The frequency of feeling of numbness is an indication of altered peripherel nerve function.

What type of desire phase disorders develop?

In one survey 39% described being aversive to sexual interest. Sexual aversion is a distinct phobic reaction.

What is the cause of sexual change?

Common causes are –

- Slowness of vaginal lubrication.
- Less erotic response to vulvar, clitoral, breast and nipple stimulation.
- More difficulty focussing on tactile sensations.
- An increasing preference for intercourse without extensive foreplay.
- Fewer sexual fantasies and preoccupations.

What sexual anatomical and physiological changes takes place?

Ovarian failure results in decreasing blood flow. Pubic hair becomes less numerous and coarser. Labia majora shrinks so do labia minora and clitoris.

Vagina suffers more, it becomes flat, looses its rough,

rigid appearance. Depth decreases and walls become thin loosing its elasticity. Environment becomes less acidic. Uterus returns to prepubertal size. Orgasmic contraction still occurs but contractions of anus does not occur.

Rates of masturbation declines.

How physical limitations affect the sex behaviour?

Physical limitations which affect sexual performance or response force the couple to adopt other options. Often they opt for an abstinence.

What are the sociological factors?

Some of couples may loose the opportunity of having intercourse not only through the death or infirmity of one partner but due to prolonged period of abstinence also. Sexual abstinence over a long period decreases the individuals assurance of sexual capability, specially for widows or divorced women.

Excessive eating, drinking and fatigue may cause sexual deterioration.

Which medical problems bring sexual boredom?

Some menopausal females may be having concurrent medical problems. Diseases like tuberculosis may result in low sex drive. The dialysis patients functions better immediately after treatment but becomes sexually dull when need of dialysis recurs.

Older diabetic patients suffer more from low sex drive.

Can certain medicines result in loss in sexual activities?

More liberal, use of anti-cholinergics, adrenergics and beta blockers to treat hypertension, vascular diseases may affect sexual performance.

Urinary Tract Infection and Menopause

Mani Raj Sharma

What do you understand by incontinence?

In menopausal age group one of the most distressing and debilitating condition is of urinary incontinence. Female urinary tract dysfunction is a major problem.

The bladder and urethra act as a functional unit with a dual purpose.

(i) to act as a storage reservoir for urine during resting phase.

(ii) to expel urine completely under voluntary control during the active phase.

What type of clinical implication can be seen?

The most common urological complaints include –

- incontinence.
- frequency, urgency and dysuria.
- voiding difficulties.

Majority of patients present after the menopause.

What about incontinence of urine?

Many authors could not establish a clear cut relationship between incontinence of urine and menopause. Still many doctors have treated postmenopausal woman with estrogen to help the disease.

In what way urinary tract infection can be present?

Often the cardinal features are frequency, urgency and dysuria. Increased incidence may be due to a greater residental urine.

What is urethral syndrome?

Recurrent episodes of frequency and urgency with dysuria in the absence of bacteria is termed 'urethral syndrome'. It does not have a single cause.

What voiding difficulties can be met?

Poor stream, straining to void, and incomplete bladder emptying are the symptoms. Estrogen deficiency may lead to distal urethral stenosis. Estrogen supplement helps in management.

How to Select a Patient for Drug Treatment

Dr. Vandana Mangal

What is the basic concept of females?

One group of females think that menopause is a natural phenomenon and it does not require any treatment while another group thinks that menopause is due to deficiency of hormones and require treatment.

What are its acute symptoms?

These include hot flushes and night sweats. These are often accompanied by palpitation and headache. Certain psychological symptoms include anxiety, forgetfulness and difficulty in concentration.

What are intermediate symptoms?

Vagina and urethra are affected. Repeated infections may lead to fibrosis. Skin becomes thin and dry.

What are long term problems?

Post menopausal bone mass requires evaluation being decreased. Osteoporosis develops. Patients may be symptomatic or asymptomatic.

Who comes for treatment?

Patients visit doctor for night sweating disturbing sleep rhythms. Some may come due to decline in sex drive. While some educated females contact doctors to rule out osteoporosis.

What non hormonal preparations can help?

Hypnotics, sedatives and tranquillizers can relive symptoms. Clonidine may prove useful. Estrogen therapy has to be started.

Principles of Hormone Replacement Therapy

Dr. R. D. Chauhan

What do you understand by HRT?

Hormonal replacement therapy is to get relief of menopausal symptoms or for the long term benefits to the skeletal and cardiovascular systems.

The decision to start HRT or not is not always a simple one and many women find it difficult to obtain the information they need to take decision.

What is HRT

It consists mainly of two hormones, estrogen and progestogen. Out of two, estrogen is more beneficial in relieving menopausal symptoms. In presence of uterus both hormones are prescribed. Adding a progestogen either cyclically or continuously protects the endometrium from hyperplastic changes.

What type of estrogens are used?

Usually natural estrogens are used. 17-β estradiol and estriol are used in HRT. Synthetic estrogen of contraceptive pill are not used in modern time due to increased risk of thrombosis and hypertension.

How to decide which type or estrogen is to be given?

There are two choices pill or a patch. Many women prefer

pill because already they are taking either B complex/ calcium, so one more pill.

Is patch more useful?

From a medical viewpoint patch has a theortical advantage in that it allows constant absorption. Migraine patients are more classic patients and they do well with patch. Thirdly patch does not increase triglycerides as occurs with oral estrogen. Similarly diabetics are very good patch candidates.

What is oral estrogen replacement therapy?

Many estrogen tablets are available in many different concentrations. Premarin ranges from 0.3, 0.45, 0.625, 0.9, 1.25 to 2.5 mg. So patient has a great choice.

Conjugated estrogen have a longer half life.

17Beta-estradiol is readily available in several dose levels 0.5 mg, 1 mg, 1.5 mg. Most doctors prefer 0.5 mg.

What is the utility of vaginal estrogen?

Vaginal estrogen have increased in popularity. Hot flashes do tend to decrease with time but atrophic vaginal symptoms can become more pronounced.

What are vaginal estrogen creams?

These are sold in tubes with a vaginal applicator. Standard dose is 1-2 gms administered vaginally at night. Many women find that 1 gm. dose is sufficient and any amount exceeding leaks out the next morning. One should not use the estrogen cream as a lubricant for intercourse.

This cream should be applied twice a week. If patient develops irritation by this tube, brand can be changed

Can vaginal tablets be used?

Tablets show less systemic absorption than the creams. Many women prefer tablets because it is less messy. Woman has to insert tablet every night for 2 weeks initially. Most women end up using tablets 2-3 times a week. Some women use cream and tablets alternately. When vulva is atrophied only cream will be more useful.

Are rings also available?

Yes the estring, a silicone ring impregnated with estradiol which is slowly released into vagina at the rate of 7.5 µg per day is available. Ring does not interfere in intercourse. The advantage of ring is that the amount of estrogen which is systemically absorbed is practically nil. There has been no secondary shock.

What is 'Ferm Ring'?

Ferm Ring is different from Estring. It delivers estrogen transvaginally to the blood stream in levels of 0.05 mg. It improves vaginal lubrication also. But some women may not feel comfortable with inserting and taking out of ring. Its major advantage is that it needs to be changed every 3 months.

When Tamoxifen is used?

Woman with metastatic concern may use vaginal tamoxifen

for relieving atrophic symptoms and get good result. Recommended dose is one or half tablet applied vaginally twice daily.

PROGESTERONE

How was provera used?

In 1980 provera 2.5 mg was given on daily basis. Disadvantage of it was that many woman developed significant unpredictable bleeding. Patient should be told about it, in advance.

To overcome this premphase came into market. It consists of 0.625 mg. of conjugated equino estrogen taken alone daily for 14 days followed by a combined pill consisting of 0.625 mg of estrogen plus 5 mg of provera for the next 14 days. Some women may complaint of irritability and breast soreness.

TESTOSTERONE

In which cases testosterone may be given?

It needs to be administered in a transdermal, trans mucus membrane or injectable form. Orally methyltestosterone which has the potential side effect of causing liver damage.

What is the advantage of methylestosterone and estrogen?

This combination decreases the production of sex hormone binding globulin and increases effective estrogen level.

When estrogen alone is not able to control hot flushes it may be given.

In what form testosterone can be used by females?

When women use this product they should apply no more than a quarter of 2.5 gm packet daily and apply it to lower part of abdomen.

Why Some Women do not go for Hormone Therapy

Dr. Rati Acharya

Still many of women do not go for HRT (Hormonal Replacement Therapy). Hardly 35% Indian well educated females undergo HRT and out of these about 50% leave after a year. Actually even most of educated females do not take menopause as a medical condition. For them it is an old age sequence and is a natural process.

What are the common reasons to not to choose hormones?

Common reasons are –

(i) Most of woman see menopause as a natural process. So they willingly tolerate hot flushes and mood swings.

(ii) Many women go to a doctor to simply confirm the diagnosis of menopause and a little assurance.

(iii) As regards osteoporosis ladies believe that due to an old age bones become weak. We are grateful to T.V. and publicity sections of pharmaceutical companies who have started public understanding osteoporosis and in return promoting sale of their products.

(iv) Women are generally afraid of using hormones. On the other hand women who have experienced side effects give a vast publicity making others afraid to use hormones. Menopausal women do not want to gain more weight.

(v) It is well known that good fat free diet, aerobic exercise, high fiber inclusion prevent heart diseases. Hormone supplementation is not taken as preventive measure. It may be a part of treatment only.

(vi) To start treatment one has to under go battery of tests lipid profile, tendency of blood clot, fibroids and mamogram to rule out any pathology of chest. So many regular tests creates a doubt about the safely of hormone treatment.

(vii) Ladies are afraid of breast cancer developed due to extended use of hormone therapy.

(viii) Estrogen therapy may give quality life but does not prolong life.

Risk Factors of Hormonal Replacement Therapy

N. K. Goyal NML

What are the chances of breast cancer?

Breast cancer is the most common complication of HRT. Otherwise also early menarche, late menopause, delayed child bearing and nulliparity is associated with higher risk of breast cancer. Post menopausal women with high oestradiol concentrations are at increased risk.

Is BMI and body weight have any relationship of developing cancer?

There is relative increase in breast cancer associated with long duration of use with a BMI of less than 25 kg/m^2. Consumption of alcohol does not affect it.

There is no increased risk of breast cancer in women taking. HRT who had already a history of benign proliferative breast disease.

How to classify risk of breast cancer?

- Short term use of HRT of less than 5 years is not associated with increased risk of breast cancer.
- Estrogen and progestin trial increases risk after 4 years of use.
- Longer use of more than 5 years of HRT increases the risk of breast cancer.

Incidence of developing breast cancer increases but not the mortality rate.

What about endometrial cancer?

Estrogen therapy increases the risk of developing both endometrial hyperplasia and endometrial cancer in post menopausal women with uterus. The relative risk of endometrial cancer in women using estrogen compared to non users is 2.3. The risk remains elevated to 5 or more years after discontinuation of estrogen.

How much is the risk of endometrial hyperplasia?

There is more conclusive evidence of effects of combined therapy to develop endometrial hyperplasia. Endometrial cancer has traditionally been considered contraindication to HRT.

Can HRT produce ovarian cancer?

The effect of HRT is unclear. If HRT is used for more than 10 years then it increases the risk of developing ovarian cancer. Risk appears largely confined to estrogen and sequential use of progestin. Treatment includes bilateral salpings-oophorectomy.

Can HRT result in venous thromboembolism?

The pathophysiology of estrogen induced VTÉ is not well understood. Oestrogen has effects on vascular endothelium and on coagulation factors that may influence VTE. It is mostly seen in –

- Hip or lower limb fracture.
- Cancer.
- Surgery.
- Late onset of menopause after the age of 52+.

Section II

Male Menopause

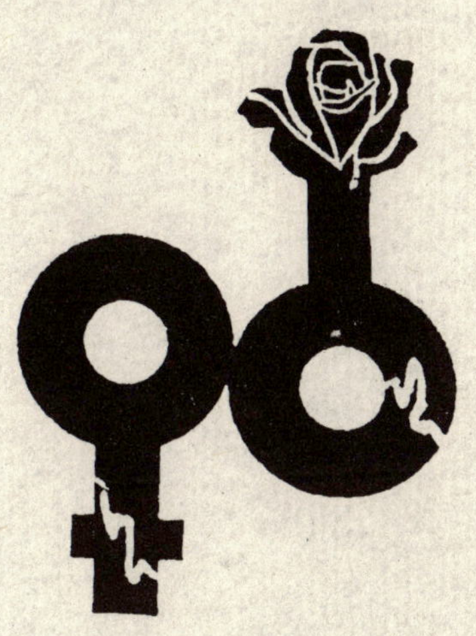

Anatomy of Male Genitals

Dr. L. C. Gupta

Are man and woman different?

Actually men and women have identical anatomical structures for the first 6 weeks of pregnancy and are born

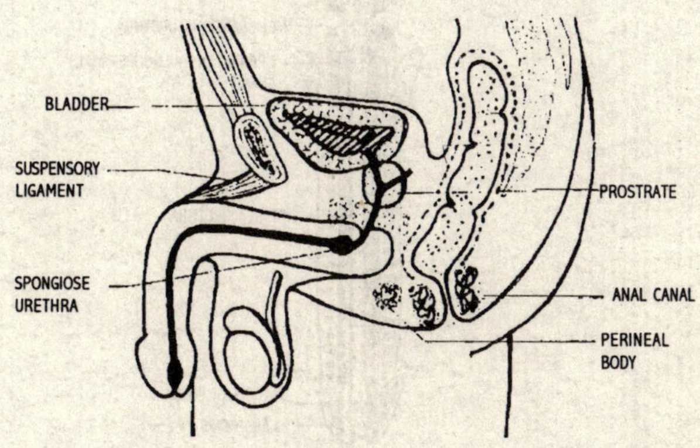

MALE PELVIC ORGANS

and developed in the same environment still they differ dramatically. Man may not be superior or inferior. Still this is a man who becomes woman's life mate. It is with man only that woman faces joys and challanges of life.

How one can understand male's sexuality?

To understand male sexuality one has to know about his sexual anatomy. After knowing anatomy only one can make

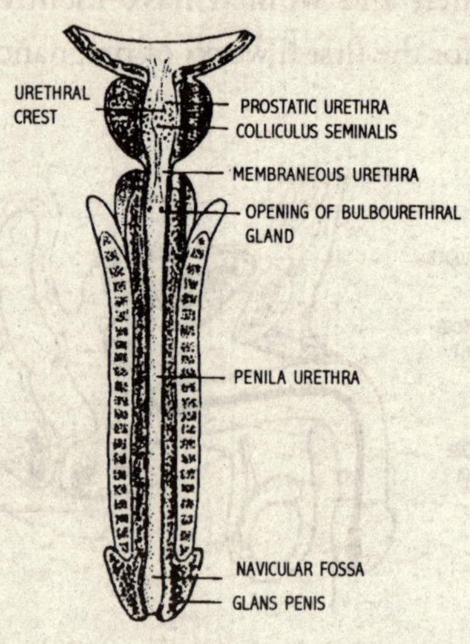

better sense of how they respond and work together in sexual situation.

What is the anatomy of penis?

This is the epicenter of man's sense of manhood. It is a symbol of potency and sexuality too. Penis has two functions –

(i) It passes out urine from bladder.

(ii) It delivers semen to a woman's womb.

The shaft of penis consists of three tubes of cylinders. Two of them are resting on the top of third. Upper ones are known as cavernous cavernosa and bottom one is known as corporus spongiosa.

Urethra runs through the bottom tube from one end to another one.

Each tube consists of spongy tissue and small smooth muscles. They are wrapped in an elastic sheath known as tunica albuginea.

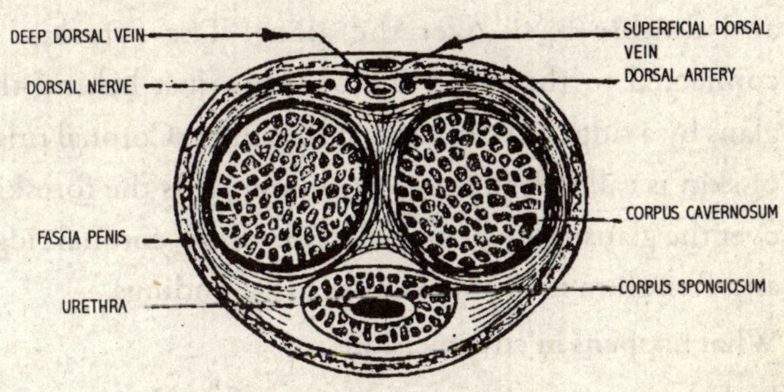

TRANSVERSE SECTION OF PENIS

What happens during arousal?

When penis is aroused, the coroporal bodies become engorged with blood. Tunica albuginea surrounding the bottom tube is thinner than that of upper corporal bodies. When erect, the bottom tube is not as rigid as upper tubes.

End of corpus spongiosum extends over the upper tubes and forms the head of the penis, known as glans penis. During erection it becomes too much engorged and grows larger in size. It becomes purplish in colour remaining soft and spongy. At the tip of glans is an opening known as meatus.

What is circumscision?

The place where skin of penis meets the glans is known as coronal ridge. In new born skin extends from the coronal ridge forward to cover the glans. It folds over and double back over the glans. The foreskin is connected to the underside of penis, just behind the glans by a ridge of skin kown as frenulum. Coronal ridge of skin is called frenulum. Frenulum pulls the foreskin over the glans when penis is flaccid. Glans, coronal ridge and frenulum have many more nerve endings.

What happens in circumcision?

In this minor operation the folded over foreskin is cut away just beyond the coronal ridge, leaving the glans penis exposed. It decreases the chances of developing infection.

What about the size of penis?

The average length of flaccid penis is between three and a half to four inches; size of flaccid penis depends on external temperature, mood and even body weight.

Does size of penis makes any difference?

Size does not make any difference but this is not totally true. It is true that outer 2.5 inches of vagina only has nerve endings which is sensitive. Rest length of penis is not felt by vagina, how so ever bigger it may be. Some women are not able to enjoy sex because of excessive girth of penis. For them size of penis makes a difference but unfortunately negative one.

Size also makes a positive difference for some females. They enjoy the feeling of containing a penis that stretches the vaginal opening. They report that they like to feel penis "filling them up." In addition to girth of penis, the length of the penis makes a difference for some women who enjoy when a penis is long enough to stimulate the cervix directly.

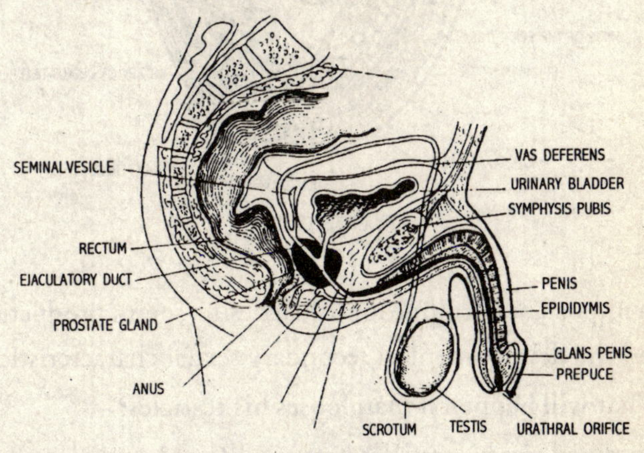

MALE REPRODUCTIVE ORGANS

What is scrotum?

It is a pouch of loose, wrinkled skin lined by tunica dartos. Hanging below penis scrotum has two compartments one for each of testicles.

What is the role of testicles?

Testicles are oval glands measuring about an inch wide. Testicles produce testosterone and sperm. Testosterone is

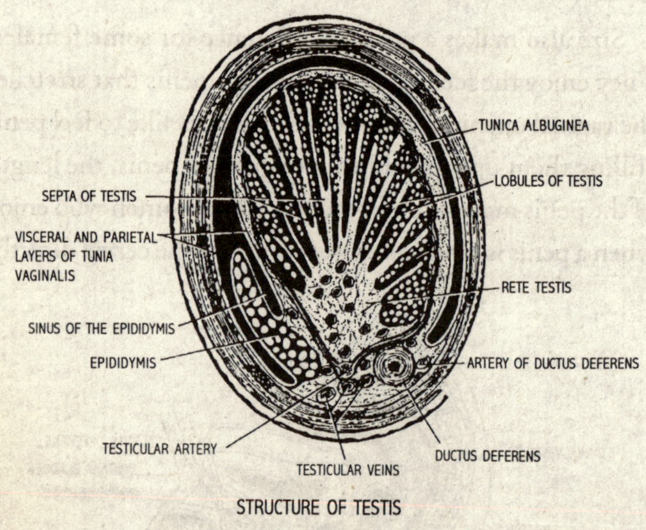

STRUCTURE OF TESTIS

an important hormone for sexual desire, sperm production and the development of secondary sexual characteristics.

What will happen if man looses his testicles?

If a man loses his testicles before puberty he will be sterile as an adult. He will likely have little interest in sex. Face hair will be thin and sparse. Damage of testicles after puberty can lead to reproductive problems.

What are sperms?

Starting from puberty sperm production remains continuous throughout life. 50,000 are produced at every minute. It takes 70 days for sperm to mature fully.

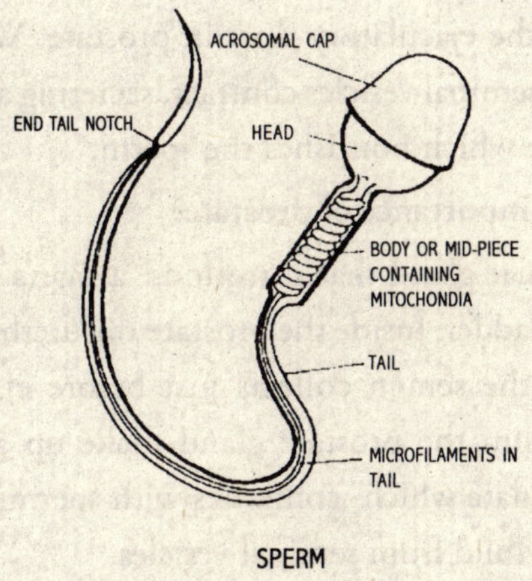

SPERM

On the upper back surface of testicle lies epididymis. Once sperm are manufactured sperm move for storage and maturation to epididymis.

When man becomes sexually aroused as many as 500 million mature sperms are moved through vas deferens.

Why sperms are stored in epididymis?

Sperm need to be manufactured and stored at about 2 degrees lower than normal body temperature. Sperm cannot survive very long at normal body temperature.

What are seminal vesicles?

There are 2 seminal vesicles small in size located behind bladder. Opening of this gland joins with vas deferens and connects to the ejaculatory duct in prostate. When man orgasms the seminal vesicles contract, secreting a fluid rich with fructose which nourishes the sperm.

What is the importance of prostate?

It is a muscular gland that surrounds a man's urethra at the base of bladder. Inside the prostate the urethra forms a bulb where the semen collects just before ejaculation. Secretions from the prostate gland make up about one third of ejaculate which combines with sperms from vas deferens and fluid from seminal vesicles.

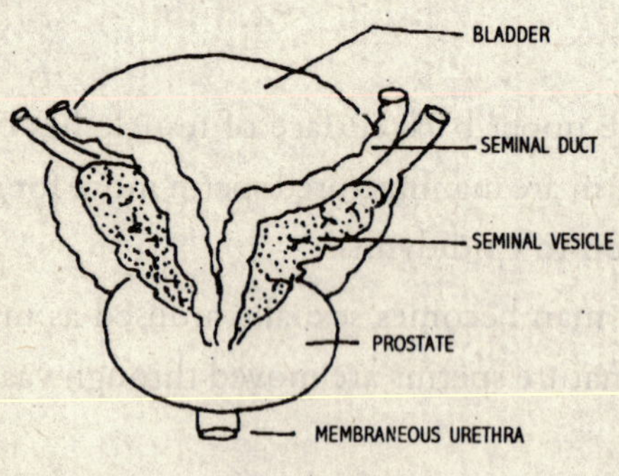

PROSTATE GLAND

What will happen if prostate is surgically removed?

If prostate is surgically removed a man will be able to experience an orgasm but he will not ejaculate. With the removal of prostate, vas deferens and seminal vesicles no longer connect to urethra. Hence prostatic fluid, seminal fluid and sperms are no longer available to create ejaculate.

What is the role of cowper's glands?

These are two small glands that connect to urethra below the prostate. During sexual arousal these glands secrete a mucous substance into the urethra which protects the sperm cells by neutralizing any acidity that may remain in urethra of earlier urination. Discharge from cowper's glands also serves as a lubricant for glans penis.

What will happen if the ovary is surgically removed?

If prostate is surgically removed a man will be able to experience an orgasm but he will not ejaculate. With the removal of prostate, vas deferens and seminal vesicles [illegible] [illegible] [illegible]. Hence, a prostatic fluid, seminal fluid and sperms are not [illegible] available to create ejaculate.

What is the role of cowper's glands?

These are two small glands that contribute to urethra below the prostate. During sexual arousal these glands secrete a mucous substance into the urethra which protects the sperm [illegible] by neutralizing any acidity that may remain in the urethra after urination. Sometimes, from cowper's glands [illegible] [illegible] for [illegible].

Male Menopause Fact or Fiction

Dr. Abhitabh Gupta & Dr. U. C. Sahu

Is male menopause term appropriate?

Generally menopause suggests a sudden drop in sex hormones which does not occur in case of males.

Is male climacteric term more suitable?

During earlier century the term male climetric (from the kilimacter – the rung of ladder) was used and seems to be more appropriate as it suggests a decline and not a precipitous drop in hormone concentration. But owing to the similarity between most of symptoms in men and women the term menopause gained popularity.

Can such symptoms may be simply due to an old age?

Ageing is usually associated with hypotestosteronaemia; depressed mood may be due to low concentration of bioavailable testosterone in older man.

Male ageing is associated with an increase in central and upper body fat deposition and reduced muscle mass and strength. It is due to age related decline in growth hormone which itself is associated with an increase in sex hormone binding globulin and therefore a reduction in bioavailable testosterone.

What other terms have been suggested?

Symptoms experienced by aged males are nonspecific and

some may be similar of hypogonadism. Therefore it is suggested that slightly decreasing testosterone levels may be accountable for some of these symptoms. In line with this hypothesis the term 'Andropause' has been suggested for men. Although no accurate definition for this term exist.

Alternating names for 'Andropause' has been suggested for men includes –

(i) Mid life crisis.

(ii) Male menopause.

(iii) Androgen deficiency in ageing males (ADAM).

(iv) Partial androgen deficiency in ageing males (PADAM).

What confusions exist?

According to some studies there is no significant association between endogenous testosterone levels and 'andropausal symptoms' in a healthy male population. Moreover no definite option exists on the cut off values for testosterone beyond which therapy should be started and it is not clear if total or free testosterone are to be measured at all.

Unlike in women where the presence of regular menses indicates normal gonadal function, we have no specific clinical criteria in men to define normal and abnormal state.

What important points are there to evaluate male menopause?

Factors that may confound diagnosis of andropause are –

- Chronic illness i.e. diabetes, renal failure and cirrhosis.
- Clinical depression.
- Decrease in albumin from alcohol abuse and poor nutrition.
- Hypothyroidism and Cushing's syndrome.
- Circadian rhythm of testosterone.

What laboratory investigations are useful?

Thorough history should be taken before reaching a provisional diagnosis of male menopause. Radioimmuneassay remains the most standard method of assessing testosterone. Saliva testing for testosterone is a novel and convinient method. If this test is done correctly, results correlate well with free testosterone levels.

Free testosterone levels of 50 mg/L or total testosterone levels of less than 260 ng/dl with consistent clinical symptoms are diagnostic of androgen deficiency. Although testosterone is secreted in spurts and the levels are highest after awakening, the daily fluctuation in serum testosterone level is attenuated in older men.

What other tests should be done?

If the testosterone level is low, further evaluation should

be done to know whether there are reversible causes of low testosterone level. Leuteinizing (LH) and follicle stimulating hormone should also be measured. Some men may show slight rise in LH level. Rise is modest compared to menopause.

Because there may be overlapping conditions giving impression of andropause syndrome it will be reasonable to measure thyrotropin and cortisol level.

Testosterone

Dr. Rajneesh & Dr. Abhishek

What is testosterone?

It is a 19 carbon steroid secreted by the testis. It directly or indirectly affects the body system. In man 3-10 mg testosterone is secreted daily by testis. Leydig cells are mainly responsible for it.

Why level of testosterone in old age falls down?

Cause of falling level is multifactorial –

(i) There is decline in leydig cell mass.

(ii) Dysfunction of hypothalamic pituitary homeostatic control.

(iii) Low lutenizing hormone secretion.

What are the other factors to lower down testosterone level?

Testosterone and free testosterone levels are sensitive to a wide range of other etiological factors. Factors include –

(i) Testicular trauma.

(ii) Physical and psychological stress.

(iii) Obesity.

(iv) Chemo and Radiotherapy.

(v) Alcohol abuse.

(vi) Malnutrition.

and any chronic disease can all adversely affect testosterone levels.

What is the significance of low testosterone level?

Low testosterone levels have been shown to be a risk factor for coronary atheroscelorisis and myocardial infarction through disturbance of blood clotting. Low testosterone levels are also associated with other risk factors such as type 2 diabetes, obesity and hypertension.

What are the normal levels of testosterone?

Mean plasma sex hormone levels in healthy men.

Age	Testosterone (n mol/L)	Free testosterone (n mol/L)	Sex hormone binding globulin (n mol/L)
25-34	21.38	0.428	35.5
35-44	23.14	0.356	40.1
45-54	21.02	0.314	44.6
55-64	19-49	0.288	45.5
65-74	18.15	0.239	48.7
75-84	16.32	0.207	51.7

What are the symptoms of hypotestosterenemia?

Frequent features are –

- Loss of libido.

- Erectile dysfunction. Difficulty in maintaining erection.
- Diminished early morning erection.
- Increased sweating, night sweats.
- Fatigue and lassitude.
- Anxiety.
- Depressed mood.
- Loss of interest in life. Loss of drive and enthusiasm.

What are the occasional symptoms of low testosterone?

Occasional features are –

- Disturbed sleep pattern.
- Loss of sensitivity of erogenous zones.
- Cold and shrivelled penis.
- Weight gain and difficult to loose it.
- Reduced seminal volume.
- Reduced orgasmic sensation.
- Dry skin.
- Reduced facial hair growth.
- Reduced volume of testis. There may be pain.
- Urinary frequency, urgency and nocturia.

Is there any relationship between testosterone and Alzheimer's disease?

Evidence is emerging that supplementation of low testosterone levels could be protective against Alzheimer's disease.

Fatigue, Irritability

Decreased muscle mass

Loss of memory, of cognitive functions

Cold and clammy skin

Weight gain and difficulty in losing it

Reduced testicular volume

Reduced armpit hair growth

Male Sexual Response

Dr. S. K. Acharya
Dr. Rati Acharya

Before knowing the effect of testosterone on sex and sexual response it is necessary to understand the physiology of sexual response in detail, male sexual response, arousal and orgasm.

What do you understand by desire?

To have desire is the starting point. To have sex man needs to want sex. Men unlike woman can become aroused and orgasm without much of sexual desire, but the presence or absence of desire will greatly influence sexual frequency and satisfaction.

Frequency of sexual thoughts and fantansies depends on rise and fall of testosterone level. If this hormone level is below normal he may miss the woman's invitating cue.

Is there a gender difference in sexual desire?

It is not true. Both women and men are capable of having strong drives. It is not the biology but our culture conditions that makes women and men act differently. Most men for example have been programmed to interpret having sex as the ultimate evidence of their desirability and masculanity. On the other hand sex can be great, but for women it's not as critical an ingredient for making an event or special as it is for most men. Sexual attention for woman may not always be a sign of affection. For many women, being held, respected and listened to are sex-signal that they are special, cherished and desired.

What do you understand by arousal?

During this stage blood enters into corporal bodies of penis. When man becomes sexually aroused impulses are sent along parasympathetic nerve fibres in penis and releases GMPA chemical which relaxes the smooth muscles. As a result pockets are formed and blood quickly pours in. Spongy tissue expands and spaces are filled with blood. As a result man has a rigid erection.

If the arteries are blocked blood will not flow in quickly enough to create the pressure necessary for erection. If the veins leak still erection will not sustain for long.

What other changes takes place in body during arousal?

While penis is in process of becoming erect a number of additional changes takes place. Breathing, heart rate and blood pressure all increases. Blood flow to skin may result in sex flush affecting earlobes, lips and nipples. Testicles become engorged and increases in size. Scrotal skin thickens and contracts. Sometimes a drop or two of a clear, slippery fluid from cowper's glands appears at the urethral opening.

What is an emission phase of an orgasm?

Male orgasm consistss of two phases. One is an emission follwed by expulsion of semen.

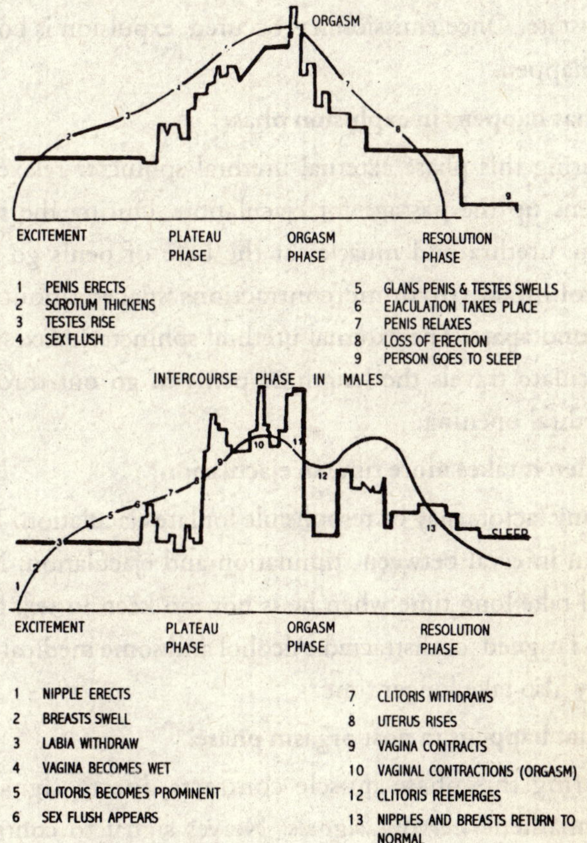

Emission of phase starts when sexual arousal reaches at maximum. There develops a series of contractions in vas deferens, seminal vesicles and prostate gland. These force semen to urethral bulb. Urethral bulb is located in the prostate. Once emission has occured, expulsion is bound to happen.

What happens in explusion phase?

During this phase external urethral sphincter relaxes. It opens up the passage for ejaculation. During the same time urethra and muscles at the base of penis go into involuntary, rhythmic contractions spaced about 0.8 second apart. The external urethral sphincter relaxes and ejaculate travels the length of penis to go out through urethral opening.

When it takes more time in ejaculation?

Many factors may be responsible for late ejaculation. That is an interval between stimulation and ejaculation. Man will take long time when he is not too keen in sex, he is too fatigued, or distracted. Alcohol and some medications may also take longer time.

What happens in post orgasm phase?

During this phase muscle contracts due to signal of sympathetic nervous signals. Nerves signal to contract. Enzymes are relaxed to break down the cyclic GMP the chemical that relaxes the muscles. Muscles relax and pressure – squeeze on the outgoing veins is released. As a result penis becomes flaccid again.

What is a refractory period?

When blood flow is reversed following orgasm, man enters into a refractory period. It is a period of time when body is not capable of rearousal and orgasm. This period is very short for young men and increases with age. It may extend from hours to days to get further erection.

Does an old age decreases sexual drive?

During young age sex is always in their mind. They will like to initiate lovemaking every chance they get. During his 30's man still have strong sex drives. But the novelty of sex begins to wear off due to job and family responsibilities. By late 40's and early 50's men find that their sexual desire is slowing gradually due to decreasing levels of testosterone.

Are psychological factors also responsible for decreasing sex desire?

Growing old become distressful due to presence of wrinkles, graying hair, protruding bellies and reading glasses. But physical changes alone do not seem to have big load on man's sexual desire. Whereas "woman needs to be felt desirable to feel sexual desire."

Man being active partner in sex avoids sex to avoid potential humiliation of erectile failure. In the bargain they loose emotional intimacy with their partner.

Why it takes longer to get erection?

Teenagers try to keep their erections down while the problem of an old age is to get erection even on effort. This change in old age is natural and it should not interfere in lovemaking with co-operative wife.

How fiction or friction can help in old age?

Fiction means having sexy thoughts and nature takes its own course. Friction refers to the direct stimulation of penis by himself or by partner. Stopping of direct stimulation will let down erection. But if the man does not panic erection will typically come back.

What types of erections are there?

It may be of 2 kinds, rock hard and rigid. In old age every thing vanishes but still will be able to become sufficiently erect to enter vagina. Angle of erection may be lesser than young age.

Why it takes longer to ejaculate in old age?

Young man ejaculate very rapidly. With age and increased sexual experience they are able to last longer. Some may take so long to ejaculate that on occasion they will be satisfied before having even an orgasm. Women may tolerate because she is not accostomed to have an orgasm everytime she indulge in sex but man finds it difficult to accept failure and even avoid lovemaking altogether rather then going through frustration of not ejaculating.

How character of ejaculation changes with age?

After the age of 30's man will begin to notice changes in his ejaculation. Generally amount of ejaculate, force of expulsion and number of muscular contractions decrease with age. Sometimes only a few drops of semen may dribble.

Is detumescence quicker in older age group?

After an intercourse a young man may remain in partner's vagina for minutes enjoying the few additional movements of physical closeness in her post orgasmic glow. While an old man may find his soft penis slipping out immediately after ejaculation. He can only hold and caress her.

Is there any positive change in man's sexual response in old age?

Yes, men in longer relationship become more comfortable with physical and emotional intimacy. They become sensitive lovers. They become much more responsive to touch.

SEXUAL DYSFUNCTIONS

Problems of sexual dysfunction may not be life threatening but they diminish the quality of life. They do not go to doctors and feel embarrassment expressing their sexual problem to a doctor. All doctors are also not knowledgeable.

What type of erectile dysfunction may take place?

Erectile dysfunction or impotence is the inability of man to get erection for satisfactory penetration of vagina. Flaccid and soft penis although adequate to pass out urine is unable to penetrate. It may be of two types, arteriosclerotic or venogenic.

What happens in arteriosclerotic impotence?

Arteriosclerosis results in stenosis and does not permit sufficient blood into erectile tissues of penis. For this penile blood pressure index, penile blood flow measurement and selective pudendal arteriography helps. Corrective revascularization surgery is useful.

How venogenic impotence develops?

Leakage of blood from the corpus cavernosum through the penile vein may result in impotence. It may be seen in abnormally large veins. Poor inflow of arterial blood may also result it because it remains unfit to block venous blood. Fibrous replacement of cavernosum may also result it. Ligation on venous leakage may help.

Can there be neurogenic impotence?

It may result due to spinal cord injury, multiple sclerosis or diabetic neuropathy.

What are the causes of organic impotence?

Excessive smoking, alcoholism, hypertension, fatigue, general debility or surgery may contribute to organic impotence. Psychological impotence develops at once. Initial failure results in further failure.

How to diagnose psychogenic impotence?

A postive nocturnal erection indicates that patient is suffering from psychogenic impotence. Secondly if patient can achieve full erection during masturbation or with different lady then he is a case of psychogenic impotence.

Full erection after I. V. injection of 10 microgram prostaglandin E1 with in 10 minutes of injection is an indication of psychogenic impotence.

What about loss of desire?

Man wants sex. It is only woman who gets headache to avoid sex. Still both sexes can develop loss of desire. Testosterone supplements can help.

What are androgen's effects on sexual function?

Primary interest on sex and its motivation depends on testosterone. It regulates libido than erectile function. Testosterone replacement in young, androgen dificient man improves a wide range of sexual behaviour including sexual desire, spontaneous erections, episodes of nocturnal erections and duration of penile erections in response to visual erotic stimuli. Penile rigidity may require physiological testosterone concentractions. Only 8-10% of men presenting with erectile dysfunction have low estrogen level.

Testosterone administration does not improve sexual function in impotent men with normal testosterone level.

What about the desire for sex?

Sexual desire seems to decline with aging. Hormonal changes at menopause can dampen desire because of discomfort of dealing with the symptoms and because of reduced estrogen and androgen.

To overcome females may take time for sexual fantasy and masturbation.

Do menopausal females get sufficient arousal?

Sexual changes following menopause are often most obvious during arousal phase. The mucous membrane tissue of the vagina and part of vulva may have become thin and prone to irritation and minor injury. Lubrication during menopause and after it decreases, so lady may not enjoy sex. More over tissues become susceptible to damage from vigorous sexual activity. Liberal use of saliva can be helpful to protect against irritation and dryness.

What type of orgasms are being enjoyed by menopausal females?

It is a well known fact that regular sexual activity and orgasm help maintain a woman's sexual health. Woman who masturbates or have regular sex with a partner actually continue to lubricate more rapidly and have more estrogens circulating in the body. As regards sex proverb is "Either use it or loose it."

Kegel exercises – squeezing and relaxing the pelvic muscles can promote strength of pelvic muscles.

Yoga and Sexual Health

Dr. L. C. Gupta

Physiological factors which enhance sexual fitness are energy, good muscle tone, supple limbs and joints and efficient function of nervous system. Yoga practice promotes all of these factors.

How yoga helps?

Orgasm, is triggered off by mounting physiological excitement-pulse rate, B.P. and breathing. All accelerate during foreplay, eventually bringing climax.

With yoga one can develop mind body mastery to a high degree. Respiratory regulation is the centre of practice of yoga. Yoga brings calming effect of slow smooth breathing on body. The man who gets early orgasm should learn to stay still and breath quietly.

For women the main problem is of achieving an orgasm. Relaxation of breathing, musculature and mind keeps away the kind of psycho sexual tension that miliates against sexual fulfilment.

How abdominal retraction exercise helps?

It helps influencing upon sexual health and vitality. It also tones up the muscles of pelvic floor, relieves conjestion and activates circulation of genital area.

Can contraction of penile muscle help in erection?

Penis responding to sexual excitement engorges with blood, lifts and rises to an angle. Normally erection of penis does not come under conscious control but penile muscles of erection can be contracted, toned and strengthened. Result will be short quick 'jerk' visible in erect penis. Make ten contraction without pause. Relax a few seconds and repeat again.

Can contraction of penile muscles of ejaculation be exercised?

Ejaculatory muscles can be exercised. When passing urine, cut off the flow abruptly by conscious command, releasing the stream of urine after stopping for 5 seconds. This is to be done repeatedly till bladder is emptied.

How contraction of pelvic floor can be useful?

Hold each contraction strongly for six seconds. Five successive contractions is sufficient. This we have to learn.

Will contraction of vaginal muscles be useful?

In contracting the pelvic floor, vaginal muscles, hold contractions strongly for six seconds. It will increase flow of blood strengthening neuromuscular control.

Senses in Old Age

Dr. L. C. Gupta

Of all our senses the sense of touch is the one that is important in all intimate encounters.

How many senses work during intimacy?

Of the 5 commonly known senses, sight, smell, hearing, taste and touch – the most valuable sexual experience is of touch. When one partner touches the other, the manner in which the contact is made can express many things.

How touch helps in old age?

The stroking of partner involves not only friction but also gives the feeling of form as the hand follows the curves and countours of the body of partner.

A caress is affectionately reassuring rather than being overtly exploratory. It is utilized to help couples break up their rigid body attitudes, to facilitate intimacy and to overcome sexual difficulty.

Touch heightens sexual pleasure and accentuates the physicality of the sex act. When two persons touch one another in a spontaneous, exploratory and tender way, a psychological intimacy is created. Closeness is fundamental to the sense of intimacy between a loving couple specially in old age.

How good fragrance can help in old age?

In terms of sex, the second most important sense is that of smell. It may be a person's visual attractiveness that initially catches our attention but during foreplay both touch and smell are more important than just vision. One can close his eyes during the sex act but one cannot avoid touching and smelling the partner.

Smell carries with it certain strong feelings. The heavy adour of musk the perfume derived from one of sex glands of musk deer is exciting to certain people.

What is the role of 'vision' in sex?

Sense of touch and smell require close contact with a partner but sight enables us to make contact even when other person is at distance.

It is believed that men are more aroused by the visual aspect of female rather than the female by the sight of male. It may be culturally induced.

Women prefer to have intercourse with the lights off or else to close their eyes during sex, while man remains eager to appreciate the curves of the female.

The sight of a beautiful attractive body facilitates contact awareness and the expression of emotions. All these factors help to create fusion within the world of love.

What type of 'sounds' help in menopause?

The importance of our sense of hearing in the sexual

encounter involves the use of words and non verbal utterances as a form of communication between the partners.

Many people like soft music in the background while making love. During the sexual act female wants to hear the appeareciative words from the male whether she has reached orgasm or not.

If one makes proper use of senses he can compensate the loss of sexual performance to some extent.

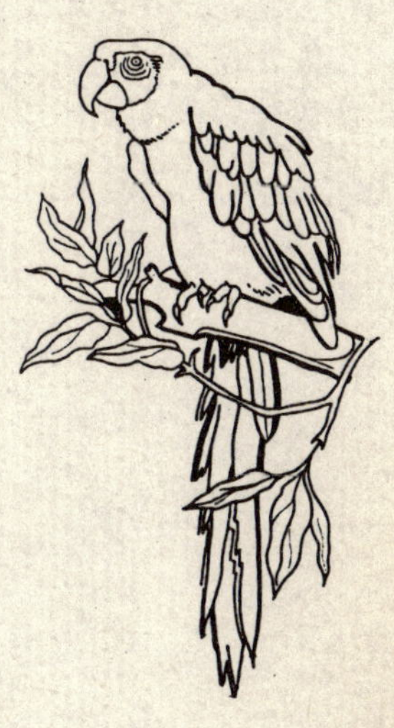

Drugs and Sex Performance

Dr. L. C. Gupta

In addition to male and female menopause certain drugs affect sex performance badly.

What is the effect of alcohol?

Every body knows that alcohol is the most common social lubricant to relieve tension and anxiety.

As blood alcohol concentration rises quickly and acutely there is likely to be an impairement of sensation, motor abilities and neural reflexes critically involved in erection and ejaculation. Chronic alcoholism is associated frequently with impotence. It seems that alcohol decreases of plasma testosterone by eliminating more of it.

What is the effect of Marijuana on sex?

It is known as a drug of considerable aphrodiasic power. Non users strongly associate marijuana with sexual persuasiveness and promiscuity amongst users. Small dose may give kick while larger doses are central nervous system depresser and depress sexuality also.

General effects of Marijuana are –

- Skin feels warm, tingly and flushed.
- Sense of touch becomes more intense and stimulating.

- Emotional warmth and affection towards one's partner appears stronger.
- Sex act appears to last longer.
- Orgasm may become more intense.

Higher doses of Marijuana may result in oligospermia and low level of testosterone.

What is the effect of sedatives on sex?

Hypnotics in old age have been misused widely to produce intoxication, general relaxation and relief of tension. Hypnotics are effective inhibitors and is followed by lethargy, loss of co-ordination and other effects. They will interfere with sexual interest.

How heroin affects one's sexual performance?

In small doses it may have push but in high doses people may complaint of reduced libido, impotency and retarded ejaculation. But these complaints are reversible with abstinence.

Withdrawl from heroin is associated with a high incidence of premature ejaculation. Serum testosterone, ejaculatory volume and sperm motility are reduced.

In younger age group it may result in amenorrhoea, infertility and reduced, libido.

How antihypertensives alter sex behaviour?

Virtually every agent used in chronic management of

hypertension has been associated with sexual dysfunction. Some of these have additional depressive effects on CNS influencing sexual behaviour.

(i) Ismelin a potent adrenergic blocker is most frequently associated with sexual dysfunction. Instances of erectile failure and loss of libido are more difficult to explain. Reserpine often not only interferes with emissions in many patients but also produces impotence and loss of libido. In young girls it can produce anovulation and amenorrhoea.

(ii) Methyldopa affects adrenergic neural transmitters and results in moderate dilatation of vessels. This drug may develop sexual dysfunction, manifested either as loss of libido, erectile failure or ejaculatory difficulties which are revealed even after two weeks of continuation.

(iii) Catapress lowers B.P. with little risk of impairing sexual function. Larger doses than 120 mg may produce impotence.

(iv) Aldactone in males is associated with estrogenic like ferminizing effects. Loss of livido and impotence are less common.

How antidepressants affect sex response?

Depression is usually accompanied with decrease in libido

and sexual activity. Due to anticholinergic effects a fair incidence of impotence and ejaculatory difficulties might be expected. Ladies have delayed orgasm.

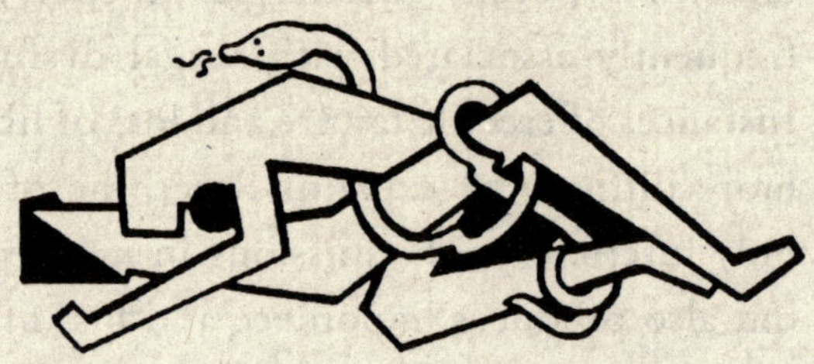

Menopause and Skin

Dr. L. C. Gupta

Educated woman is well aware of aging changes in skin. In response to their concern millions are being earned by beauty clinics. Old ladies very often visit them.

What are the common complaints?

Common complaints include wrinkles, dryness, sagging, thinning of scalp hair, increased facial hair and pigmentation.

Greatest concentration of estrogen receptors were found in face with lesser amount in breasts and thighs.

Skin collagen decreases and is due to body collagen loss and relate to lower bone collagen levels. Skin fold thickness is also decreased. Microcirculation of skin epithelium thinning and loss of tensile strength, occurs.

What other changes develop in skin?

Dry skin results from lower sweat gland response and sebaceous activity. Healing becomes slower on trauma. Depigmentation starts. 'Ageing spots' are hyperpigmentation of skin specially in fair coloured people.

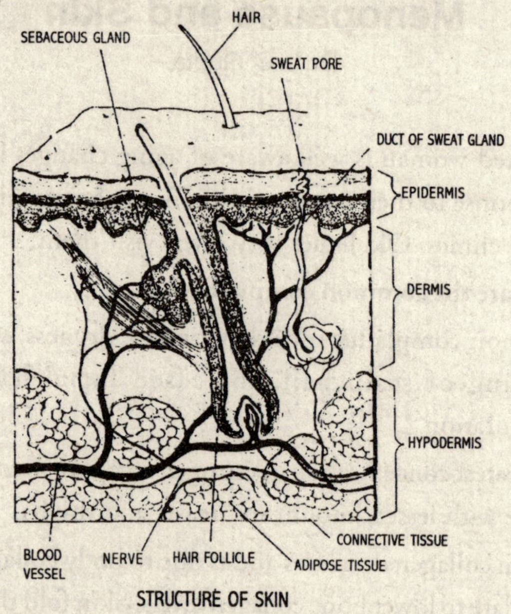

STRUCTURE OF SKIN

Some people may develop red spots. In such cases excessive exposure to sun should be discouraged.

What type of skin care is needed?

Proper nutrition is necessary. Liberal use of moisturizers prevents skin drying. Excessive exposure to sunlight should be avoided. Smoking causes hamper in microcirculation and should be discouraged.

Are estrogens helpful?

The skin absorbs estrogen rapidly. Lower doses serves the purpose. Transdermal administration of estrogen is less likely to be associated with hypertension.

How to React to Menopause

Dr. Abhishek Gupta

What are man's perception about wife's menopause?

Man feels –

- Wife is tired and irritable.
- Wife is not interested in him as she used to be.
- Interpersonal relationship is changing in uncomfortable ways.
- It is her menopause, I need not to interfere.

What is wife's perception about husband's menopause?

- Husband looks tired and irritable.
- He does not seems to be interested in me as he used to be.
- Sex has not remained enjoyable.
- He is depressed.
- Interpersonal relationship is changing in uncomfortable ways.
- He does not find me attracttive.

Is knowledge of menopause necessary?

Lack of knowledge of age related changes and hormonal influence can push relationship over edge. Neither husband nor wife will remain happy and will not be able to communicate their feelings to each other. It leads for withdrawl and isolation.

Ignorance definately is not bliss, it is a waiting disaster to happen.

How to recognise male menopause?

There is lack of definite physiological landmark as in the cessation of menses for women. Male menopause is not a disease but is a gradual change that occurs physically and emotionally between the ages of 40 and 60.

When man suffers in silence?

Man experiences a mild depression, low thyroid levels, an enlarged prostate and borderline decline in his testosterone level.

Is becoming sensitive to each others needs necessary?

One has to be a sensitive for strengthening intimacy. Actually we remain so busy in our problems that we lose sight of our partner's concern. We should listen partner with empathy and understanding. Learn yourself about what changes your partner may be experiencing affectionate to each other.

What about old anger and resentment?

If you continue to hold old grievances it will serve to erode intimacy. If past resentment surfaces, may hamper growth for a closer bond. One should acknowledge emotions of each other and start developing a fulfilling relationship.

Should there be a space between couple?

There should always be a delicate balance between being together and being apart. One should leave enough loving space for intimacy.

How to survive your husband's midlife affair?

To keep relations survive –

- Keep in mind that this situation will not last forever. There will be life after the affair and time will heal it.
- Take lead to solve problems and do not wait for husband to initiate.
- Do not retaliate.
- Surround yourself with loving environment. On occasion surrender to your husband with your body.

How husband should react with perimenopause of wife?

5 to 10 years prelude to menopause is referred as perimenopause. Actuallly this is a stage where a woman can take stock of her health, reduce her risk factors and maximize the quality of her life. Husband should be co-operative and doctor should be consulted.

How husband will recognise that wife is entering perimenopausal stage?

Following points may help –

- She is between the age of 40 and 50.

- Her periods may be regular.
- Her periods are becoming irregular.
- She has developed sleep disorder.
- Her sex drive is waning.
- She is skipping periods.

How best you can help your partner?

- Let her know about her physiological situation. Encourage her to share her feelings and needs.
- Be extra patient and kind.
- Take up healthy hobbies together.
- Give her gifts and compliments.
- Stress reduction techniques can help.

What every husband should know about his wife's menopause?

- Every woman undergoes menopause.
- Most common physical symptom of menopause is hot flush.
- Moodiness and irritability are often the effect of estrogen depletion.
- She may develop dryness of vagina and start avoiding sex.

- Certain touches which used to cause excitement may become unpleasant or uncomfortable. Wife may even develop an aversion.

What wife wants her husband to know about her menopause?

- Give her a support in life.
- I am moody, please do not take it personally.
- Let me know that you still love me. I am still important to you.
- Making me sexy is about more than sex.
- Spend at least half an hour together with me.
- Use the power of touch. Skin will release more of oxytocin and enhence your feeling of closeness.
- Share your romantic thoughts.

What every woman should know about male midlife depression?

Each wife should know that –

- Depression is the most common problem associated with male midlife crisis.
- Depression is underdiagnosed in men and over diagnosed in women.
- Feelings of sexual inadequacy can trigger depression in man.

- Excessive moodiness and irritability may be a sign of depression.
- Sleep disturbance.
- Counselling can speed recovery.
- Men have a higher risk of depression when testosterone level is low.

Testosterone Therapy

Dr. Abhishek Gupta

Testosterone supplementation can be man's best friend if he is really having a low level of testosterone. Actual decline in testosterone production with age is the result of decrease in manufacture of this hormone by the testes themselves. There becomes a loss or blunting of response to higher hormonal signals coming from brain pleading for more testosterone to be released into blood.

Morning sample of testosterone is recommended because of the known circadian rhythm in testosterone release in man. Levels of testosterone are higher in morning and can drop by 35% in afternoon and evening hours. After the age of 60 circadian nature of testosterone production is blunted and morning sample may not be necessary.

What should be the minimum level of testosterone?

If the total plasma testosterone level is less than 7.0 nm/L (200 mg/L) this is a clear indication of hypogonadism regardless of age. Thyroid disorders and pituitary tumors should be ruled out.

What to aspect after starting testosterone therapy?

Before starting the treatment evaluate the health of prostate fully for any enlargement or cancer.

Many men feel an improvement in their libido. It is accompanied by enhanced mood and overall psychological well being. It will preserve bone mass and improve lean body mass also, preventing osteroporosis.

Is testosterone helpful in reducing cardiac problems?

(i) Most studies support a corelation between higher total serum testosterone levels and lower cardiovascular diseases. It can lower total cholesterol and LDL. It has little impact on improving levels of HDL. (ii) Testosterone may act as a vasodilator, improving blood flow. (iii) Testosterone has a positive effect on mood and overall psychological well being. It can act as a mild antidepressant. (iv) It does not cause ejaculatory or impotency problems as a side effect.

What types of testosterone therapy are available?

Ideally testosterone as a supplement is a safe treatment. It is convinient, inexpensive and produce physiological levels to correct the clinical deficiency.

Testosterone is available in oral, injectable, transdermal and implantable formulations.

Oral forms include methyl testosterone and oxandrolone and is not very much recommended because it can damage the liver. They may also raise LDL cholesterol and decrease HDL levels.

Are injectable testosterone more suitable?

Intramuscular injections are being suited for many years.

Usually the dosage of 400 mg every 2-4 weeks are given. Recently scrotal and non scrotal patches are being used. It provides more natural levels of kestosterone.

Are testosterone implants also available?

Yes, testosterone has also been fused into pellets that can be implanted beneath the skin. It is convinient and normal range serum levels can be achieved for upto 6 month. It needs minor surgical interference.

How long testosterone therapy is to be continued?

Typically it is recommended to be continued for at least six months to one year. Person should be followed up for any adverse effect. Serum testosterone should be checked.

What are the contraindication and risks of testosterone therapy?

An absolute contraindication is presence of prostate or breast cancer. Ultrasound study should be got done for the

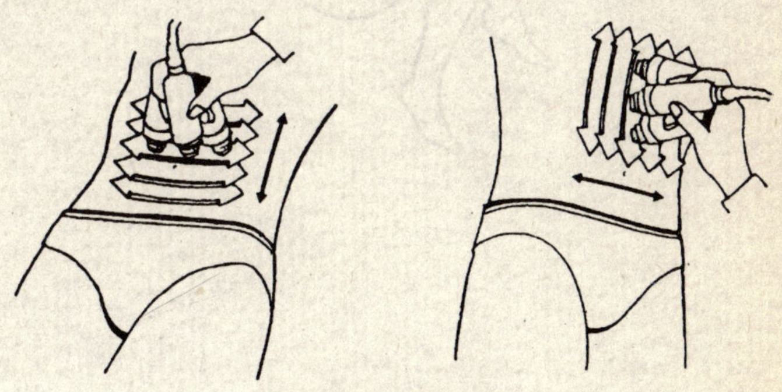

ULTRASOUND MONITORING

evaluation of prostate and breast. An androgen can promote prostate and prostatic hyperplasia.

Is testosterone for man only?

Testosterone commonly thought of as a male hormone, is also produced in women and declines significantly after menopause. A little bit of testosterone can go a long way in restoring libido, energy and mental well being. It improves sexual activity, sexual satisfaction, pleasure and orgasm when compared to estrogen therapy alone.

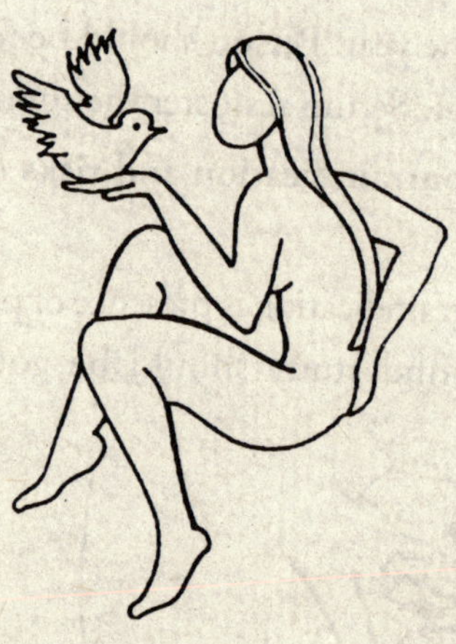